T0123122

A PATIENT-CENTERED APPROACH TO MEDICINE FOR THE TERMINALLY-ILL

Irene S. Switankowsky

University Press of America,® Inc.
Lanham · Boulder · New York · Toronto · Plymouth, UK

Copyright © 2012 by
University Press of America,® Inc.
4501 Forbes Boulevard
Suite 200
Lanham, Maryland 20706
UPA Acquisitions Department (301) 459-3366

Estover Road
Plymouth PL6 7PY
United Kingdom

Library of Congress Control Number: 2010936058
ISBN: 978-0-7618-5338-1 (paperback : alk. paper)
eISBN: 978-0-7618-5339-8

Contents

Chapter 1

Introduction

The medical literature on euthanasia is replete with cases of abuse towards terminally-ill patients. For example, sometimes, relatives want to hasten a patient's death because they believe that his/her quality of life will continue to deteriorate. Most patients would like to have a chance to give an informed decision for or against a medical procedure; however, patients and physicians have no consistent monitoring devices to help facilitate this process. The purpose of this book is to remedy this defect in medical practice by presenting a patient-centered approach of informed consent that is specifically applicable to the terminally-ill. Generally, the patient-centered approach promotes patient autonomy by developing a situation in which the physician conceives of the patient's medical situation through that patient's unique perspective.[1] I will argue that it is possible for a terminally-ill patient to give an informed consent about end-of-life issues if (s)he follows the five conditions outlined in Part II which are meant to provide a type of monitoring system, both for patients and physicians, to test the genuineness of their medical decisions. Further, these conditions can help physicians develop an open and honest relationship with their patients which is the foundation of any patient-centered approach. As Peabody reminds us,[2] the secret of effective patient care is in genuinely caring for the patient which presupposes that the physician carefully listens, considers, and reflects on the terminally-ill patient's medical and personal concerns before and during his/her illness.

To this end, the book will be divided into three main parts. In Part I, I present a characterization of the patient-centered approach and juxtapose it with a strictly physician-centered approach. In the process, I show why a patient-centered approach is necessary if a patient is to provide an informed consent for end-of-life issues since (s)he must decide upon his/her medical and personal preferences with respect to certain diseases. A patient's beliefs and values must be central to such decisions since the patient should ultimately decide how and under which circumstances (s)he will end his/her life. In Chapter 2, I will examine two main types of physician-patient relationship. In Chapter 3, I discuss the parameters of a strictly physician-centered approach and some of its difficulties, given the patient-centered paradigm to be developed in Part II of the Book. In Chapter 4, I will discuss the patient-centered model and show why this model is most beneficial in dealing with end-of-life care. Though many medical theorists believe that the patient-centered approach is opposed to the biomolecular revolution, I believe that the two approaches are compatible and can complement one another.

The biomolecular paradigm presupposes not merely improved medical knowledge but also improved physician-patient relations. In other words, the physician cannot effectively apply the new paradigm of medicine without developing an open, honest relationship with the terminally-ill patient, effectively communicating, sharing authority and decision-making, understanding the patient's experience of illness, preparing advanced directives with the terminally-ill patient, and ensuring that the terminally-ill patient gives an informed consent for a medical intervention.

In Part II, I outline five patient-centered conditions for achieving an informed consent: (1) effective disclosure; (2) successful decision-making; (3) effective communication; (4) developing an effective physician-patient relationship; and (5) preparing advance directives. These five conditions will ensure that irrationalities and biases do not occur as often in medical situations when a patient has negative perceptions of him/herself because of his/her terminally-illness. Further, being in constant pain can negatively influence a patient's attitude towards his/her overall prognosis and view of life. If these negative feelings continue to develop, they will seriously bias the patient's decision-making processes in favour of ending his/her life even though there may be other alternatives available to that patient. If a physician adheres to these guidelines, the terminally-ill patient will be able to give an informed consent for any medical procedure.

There is much abuse when it comes to deciding whether or not a terminally-ill patient should end his/her life. There are issues surrounding whether relatives should be able to decide to end a patient's life. There are also questions about whether and for how long a terminally-ill patient can make a rational and autonomous decision about end-of-life issues on his/her own. These are all complex questions for which multifaceted answers must be given. In this book, I argue that a patient's medical practitioner is the most important person to ensure that the patient will give a rational and autonomous decision about what should be done to alleviate the pain and suffering of a medical condition. I will also argue that relatives are not in any privileged position to help the terminally-ill make decisions about end of life issues. Proxy consent is riddled with difficulties and psychological complexities and living wills which are not supplemented with advance directives are especially problematic. Thus, certain preventative measures must be in place to enable terminally-ill patients to give an informed consent for a medical treatment.

To date, there is no unbiased and objective evaluation in place to determine how a physician is to ensure that a terminally-ill patient gives an informed consent when (s)he becomes terminally-ill. In Part II, I will outline a set of conditions that are necessary for a patient to give an informed consent which includes gaining a sufficient amount of self-knowledge, developing an open, honest physician-patient relationship (ideally prior to illness), and drafting up advance directives so that the patient can ideally decide before the onset of a terminal illness how (s)he prefers to be treated.[3] The patient-centered approach is the foundation for the conditions outlined in Chapters 5 to 9. Since the patient is central in each medical interaction, (s)he should strive to make his/her own informed decisions about end-of-life issues. In other words, within the patient-centered approach to be outlined in this work, a terminally-ill patient must decide for him/herself how (s)he will proceed, given his/her medical predicament and unique experience of illness.

Chapter 10 focuses on the importance of the patient-centered approach as a way of bringing about humane health care. The five conditions discussed in Part II are a fundamental aspect of the patient-centered approach since without them, humane health care cannot take place. When a patient becomes terminally-ill, the patient-centered approach is the most effective way of bringing about humane health care since it respects a patient's autonomy and dignity. Chapter 10 redefines the patient-centered approach outlined in Chapter 3, and shows how the five conditions are foundational features of the approach. This chapter examines why the patient-centered approach is especially important for a terminally-ill patient to give an informed consent. One reason why a patient-centered approach to health care must be in place for terminally-ill patients is to avoid biases and irrationalities by either the patient or his/her relatives. Many abuses are possible when terminally-ill patients can no longer make rational decisions about medical treatments for themselves. A patient-centered approach will ensure that not as many abuses occur. If only a few abuses can be avoided, the patient-centered approach is well worth the effort it takes to bring it about and advocate it.

Chapter 2

The Physician-Patient And Patient-Centered Approaches

The purpose of this chapter is to introduce two main types of physician-patient relationship, the physician-centered and patient-centered approach, and to argue that the patient-centered type of physician-patient relationship should be developed in order for humane health care to be administered for the terminally-ill. There is a substantial amount of reported abuse with terminally-ill patients who are treated by paternalistic physicians. A lot less abuse occurs when a physician strives to develop a partnership-type relationship with the terminally-ill patient. This chapter will discuss the physician-centered approach and outline some of the features of this approach, along with the drawbacks. The main theme of this chapter is that unless a patient's autonomy is respected by developing a partner-type relationship with a physician, humane health care cannot be administered for the terminally ill.

To this end, this chapter will be divided into two parts. In Part I, I will outline five main models of the physician and patient relationship: (1) benevolent paternalism;[1] (2) the customer-salesperson model;[2] (3) the contractual model;[3] (4) the partnership model;[4] and (5) the trustee model.[5] The first three models are physician-centered models while the last two are patient-centered. The first three models are ineffective to achieve a humane type of health care for the terminally ill which respects a patient's autonomy and dignity, while the last two models are more effective in achieving humane health care. In Part II, I briefly take stock of the ramifications of a physician-centered approach discussed in the chapter.

I. Five Models of the Physician-Patient Relationship

(1) Benevolent paternalism[6] relies on the traditional physician-patient relationship as its paradigm. Under this model, physicians are obligated to act in a

loving and fatherly manner towards their patients, who are usually ill-informed and uneducated about medicine and their ailments. Under this approach, great inequalities in power between patient and physician are permitted. Physicians frequently act on the patient's best medical interests, without the patient's express permission. In others words, physicians usually take it upon themselves to directly manage the patient's overall health. The difficulty with this paradigm is that it disrespects a patient because there is no open, honest communication between the patient and physician. The patient is typically uninformed and cannot formulate ideas about the health benefits of a treatment while the physician does not have a clue about the patient's overall medical benefits since (s)he cannot discuss them effectively with the patient. Thus, this model, though perhaps an improvement over the strictly paternalistic model, does not provide the necessary care which is effective to respect a patient's autonomy and dignity.

On the traditional approach of the physician-patient relationship, patients placed ultimate trust in the physician because they lacked any kind of information about their medical condition. There are several difficulties with this type of trust. First, the trust that is given by the patient is usually blind. Therefore, a patient's autonomy is disrespected in the process since (s)he leaves the decision-making power solely in the hands of his/her physician. However, this trust is misplaced, which leads me to the second difficulty with the trust that is implicit in the traditional model. Although a physician is trusted to make major decisions about a patient's health, the physician is insufficiently informed about the patient's perception of what is valuable for his/her overall health since (s)he has never talked to the patient in any detail about these things. In other words, the physician makes decisions on behalf of a patient in ignorance of any idea of the patient's beliefs, values or overall medical goals in relation to his/her condition.

This type of criticism about the traditional model of the physician-patient relationship is still prevalent today in some circumstances. In some cases, life sustaining and life prolonging measures, such as aggressive types of chemotherapy or resuscitation in dying patients, are still used without evaluating the patient's overall well-being or talking to the patient. More recently, alternative models for the physician-patient relationship has been developed which include the patient and ensure that s(he) has a prominent place in all medical decision-making. The physician is viewed as an agent who must ensure that the patient's wishes are fulfilled and that (s)he makes an informed decision about a medical intervention. These alternative models have emerged in order to decrease the inequalities of power in the physician-patient relationship, and in support of each patient's right to self-determination.

There is one important difficulty with autonomy-based alternative models of the physician-patient relationship. Some patients are incapable of making their own autonomous decisions about their health because they are either uninformed or uneducated. This poses a difficult problem for medical professionals that want to get beyond the traditional model. Let's first consider the following example.

Sally is an 80 year old woman who goes to the physician complaining of extreme fatigue, abdominal bloating, and abdominal pain. The physician did a routine pap smear and sent her to the lab for blood tests, and also suggested that she have a colonscope and a gastrioscope. After administering these tests, the physician discovered that her pap test was abnormal, signalling cervical cancer. Sally did not understand the results of the tests that the physician discussed with her. Before sending Sally to a gynaecologist for further testing, he sent her for an abdominal ultra-sound. It was discovered that Sally had fibroid tumors in her uterus and that they were cancerous. Sally did not want to go through surgery to remove the tumors and she did not want to talk about it to the family or physician. Her Gynecologist agreed that an 80 year old woman should not have a hysterectomy. However, Sally never inquired into whether there was any other medication that she could take to shrink the fibroids or stop their growth.

Four months after her diagnosis, Sally's stool was black and she was throwing up blood. She was admitted to the hospital. They performed a gastrioscope again. Sally never mentioned anything about her fibroids.The results from the gastrioscope and the colonoscope were normal. However, when they drew blood, they discovered that her haemoglobin was below 70. They gave her a transfusion, kept her in the hospital for observations for four days, and then released her.

Six months later the same sequence of symptoms and treatments occurred. She again never mentioned anything about her fibroids as the possible cause of these symptoms.

How can an autonomy-based model be applied to Sally when she clearly cannot rationally handle her medical condition? Obviously, Sally either does not appreciate the severity of her medical situation or is in denial about it. Sally is uninformed, uneducated, and most importantly does not honestly want to know what is happening with her health. However, when Sally experiences extreme fatigue and has increasing pain, she becomes angry, disillusioned and depressed. Sally can be considered untrusting, and scared of the medical profession when it comes to having a biopsy. She will not talk to anyone about her beliefs, values, medical goals or feelings, not even her own sons or daughters-in-law. Sally's medical condition seems to be continuously deteriorating, (s)he could slip into a coma at any time.

Although there are some older patients who are in the same predicament, I will not be directly dealing with them since I do not believe that the autonomy-based model could be applied to such patients. They represent a special and very problematic category of patient that I will not be dealing with in this work. Perhaps all such patients could effectively rely on is the traditional benevolent model. If a patient could not make autonomous decisions about his/her health, the autonomy-based model of the physician-patient relationship cannot effectively apply to them. An autonomous decision is a decision that is made rationally and unbiasedly by consulting one's beliefs, values, and life plans. Therefore, an autonomous decision is not merely based on an utterance of what a patient wants to do without careful reflection of the pros and cons of the decision. Instead, an autonomous decision is a multifaceted decision that involves a patient's deeply held beliefs, values, desires, and personal and medical goals. Sally, in the above example, did not make an autonomous decision about what should be done, given her diagnosis and prognosis. Sally did not have to endure a hysterectomy or any exploratory surgeries. That decision was based on a biased and irrational decision which will lead her to needless pain and suffering. Thus, the decision was made mostly by default and framed in terms of her fears instead of on the basis of careful thought and reflection.

(2) The customer-salesperson model[7] presupposes that the role of the patient should be equated to that of a 'customer' and the role of the physician is similar to that of the salesperson. According to this paradigm, the customer is always right, and the salesperson should gladly agree with everything that the patient wants, even if this is counterproductive to the prognosis of the patient. This scenario presupposes that the patient is in charge of his/her health; however, since the patient lacks medical knowledge, his/her decision will be ineffective since a terminally ill patient's access to medical information is usually derived through the media and/or other unreliable sources. Let us consider an example to illustrate this point:

> Say, an 83 year old woman, Gladys, is suffering from Rheumatoid Arthritis. Gladys visits her rheumatologist and he suggests that she keeps taking gold treatments since it seems to be alleviating her pain. Gladys develops a pain in her shoulder and convinces herself that the gold treatments are no longer working. She talks to her hairdresser who is taking metrotrixate for the relief of her rheumatoid pain. Gladys knows nothing about the medication or its side effects but she is convinced that it will help her as much as it is helping her hairdresser. Gladys makes an appointment to see her general practitioner and says that she would like to be taken off gold treatments and prescribed metotrixate instead to alleviate her pain. The physician knows how much harder it will be on her overall system; yet, he reluctantly prescribes the medication. She keeps taking the pills but throws up blood every few months. Yet, Gladys ignores that and continues taking the pills, convinced that they are helping her with the pain. She is also convinced that her pain in the shoulder is better, although some days her pain is the same or worse then it was before she started taking metotrixate.

It seems evident from this example that, on the basis of this model, Gladys's physician felt obligated to prescribe the medication that she requested without discussing the associated risks and possible harms that are possible as a result of taking the medication. This meant that Gladys was prescribed a non-steriodal, anti-inflammatory drug when there was a very high risk of gastrointestinal bleeding. According to this paradigm, the physician should provide whatever treatment or medication the patient wants, even if the physician considers that in Gladys's particular circumstances, it is harmful, risky, and unlikely to be of much benefit to her. This model of the physician-patient relationship is just as deficient as the traditional model since it is too one-sided for it to be a rational and effective way of treating patients.

(3) The contractual model[8] attempts to balance the autonomy of both the physician and patient, mainly by laying down moral and legal rules of conduct. The moral rules tend to be implied or mutually understood but they do not take the form of a written contract. However, both the moral and legal rules are considered strictly binding, although they concur. According to this paradigm, the rules are simple stating that no treatment can be administered to a patient without his/her consent if (s)he is competent to make the decision him/herself. Also, no physician can be forced to provide medical care or treatment which he strongly believes is not in the patient's best interest. In other words, no one can pressure the physician to administer a medical treatment to a patient which (s)he feels is not in the patient's best interest. This is a really problematic model of the physician-patient relationship because it lacks balance and effective focus that it promises to provide.

More specifically, there are two major problems with the contractual model. First, the model presupposes a fundamental lack of trust for the patient. Contracts are usually established between parties who feel that they cannot trust one another. In fact, the contractual model is an attempt to decrease the need for trust on the patient's behalf. However, trust is an ineradicable feature of the physician-patient relationship. Second, this model develops an uncomfortable relationship between the patient and physician, one which undermines the patient as an autonomous individual. The model also disrespects patients and this will make a patient feel even less in control due to his/her illness. Instead of creating contracts, physicians and patients should communicate with one another openly and honestly. The contractual model hinders that substantially. Thus, the contractual model is deficient to develop a humane relationship between physician and patient. Some better models between physician and patient are more patient-centered and amenable to respecting a patient's autonomy.

(4) The partnership model[9] of the physician-patient relationship presupposes that the patient and physician enters into the relationship as equal partners. In order for the patient and physician to develop an effective relationship, they must engage in open and honest communication. This model presupposes that the physician cannot effectively treat the patient's illness without knowing a lot about the patient's beliefs, values, goals, and life plans. In addition, the patient cannot have his/her illness effectively treated without relying on a physician's medical knowledge. Thus, both the physician and patient must enter into an equal partnership since the masteries of both individuals are necessary for effective health care to occur. The patient knows his/her own life plans, values, beliefs, and priorities while the physician knows how best to administer the best type of treatment to the patient.

The goals of the partnership model is for the physician and patient to work together to treat an illness. There are several facets of the partnership model which I will be describing in more detail in Chapters 5 to 10. First, the partnership model presupposes that the patient and physician develop an open, honest relationship through which they can build trust and respect. Second, the model presupposes that the physician trusts the patient sufficiently to respect the patient's autonomy each time an important medical decision must be made. Lastly, the model reinforces the fact that both the patient and physician are responsible for decisions when they are reached. Thus, the partnership model presupposes that the patient and physician engage in shared decision making in which each fulfills his/her own unique role. This is an especially important model to develop for terminally-ill individuals.

(5) A trustee[10] is an individual who acts in the best interests of another individual when (s)he cannot act or make decisions for him/herself because of senility or death. The trustee, it is assumed, will always take into account whatever is known about the wishes of the other person, and will act in his/her best interest. The trustee must always strive to act progressively with the attitudes of compassion and beneficence, and direct care honestly towards his/her overall medical improvement. But how can we be sure that the trustee knows what is in the patient's best interest? Relatives are not always the best individuals to become the patient's trustee since they are usually unaware of the best interests of the patient in relation to his/her health. This points to one of the real difficulties with this model.

Another difficulty is that many times the patient's interests are either intentionally or unintentionally misrepresented. Relatives may sometimes, either intentionally or unintentionally, bias a patient's best interest in terms of their egoistical circumstances. Even if a relative is aware of the patient's best interests (which does not occur too often), (s)he rarely represents the patient's concerns honestly much less makes rational decisions about a medical intervention on the patient's behalf. This is especially the case for terminally-ill patients since relatives tend to bias their future medical treatments in terms of death and dying. Relatives may even feel awkward to make such decisions on behalf of their relatives without first talking to them. I believe it is best for trustees not to be related to the family since then the trustee does not have a vested interest in making decisions on behalf of the patient. I will discuss the possible abuses with proxy consent in the second part of this work.

The best candidates to serve as a trustee are individual's who are familiar with the patient's values, beliefs, life goals and desires while being appointed by the medical practitioner or physician to best represent a patient's medical interests honestly, objectively, rationally, and unbiasedly. Such individuals may be medical physicians, social workers or other medical staff. Either the patient or the physician could appoint trustees. Alternatively, the patient could appoint his/her physician as his/her trustee if (s)he chooses. The patient must choose his/her trustee unless (s)he becomes senile, is in a coma, or suddenly develops Alzeheimers. Ideally, the trustee's name should be registered in a patient's living will. This should be part of the patient's medical file should the need occur for the trustee at a later date. I will discuss living wills in more detail in Chapter 9.

II. Taking Stock - Putting Things Together

Most of the models of the physician-patient relationship outlined in Chapter 2 are physician-centered models, except for the partnership model to be discussed later. The foundation of the patient-centered model, to be addressed in this book, requires that the physician and patient become equal partners with the common goal of improving a patient's health and quality of life. The physician-centered models to be discussed in the next chapter fail to sufficiently respect a patient's autonomy or to develop a physician-patient relationship that is based on mutual trust and respect. As will become apparent, the paternalistic physician-centered paradigm must be replaced by the patient-centered model which ensures that a terminally-ill patient's life will be respected and his/her dignity and quality of life will be the physician's top priority. Only the patient-centered model can ensure that the terminally-ill patient will live his/her remaining days with the respect and dignity that (s)he deserves.

Conclusion

This chapter outlined five models of the physician-patient relationship and showed that partnership-type models are the best suited to caring for the terminally ill. In the next chapter, I examine the physician-centered approach and outline some of the difficulties with this paternalistic-type of approach when caring for terminally ill patients. This approach insists that the physician is at the forefront and central to all medical decision making. The approach disrespects a patient's autonomy since the physician decides which treatment the patient ought to be prescribed without deciding with the patient. In addition, the approach insists that a physician is the expert and his/her decision ought to be respected and followed unquestioningly. Most times, this approach does not encourage the physician to develop an open and honest physician-patient relationship. Lastly, the physician-centered approach does not insist that the physician and patient become equal partners. As I argue in the next chapter, this model disrespects a terminally ill patient's autonomy and makes humane medicine impossible to achieve.

Chapter 3

The Physician-Centered Approach

In this chapter, I will discuss some of the difficulties of the physician-centered approach in more detail. A lot more must be said about physician-centered medicine since it has been so much a part of the paternalism model and is still prevalent for the care of the terminally-ill. Unless the terminally-ill have advance directives, the physician-centered paradigm is prevalent since most times either the physical or psychological features of the illness negatively affect a patient's capability to make a rational and informed decision about his/her end-of-life issues. Some terminally-ill patients can also become senile or slip into a coma. This also reduces any chance for the patient to make an informed decision about end-of-life issues, giving the physician full responsibility for the care of the patient.

The chapter will be divided into three parts. In Part I, I will define and outline five main features of the physician-centered approach. In Part II, I will list/outline some of the key difficulties with the physician-centered paradigm for achieving humanistic medicine for the terminally-ill. In Part III, I will briefly state why the physician-centered paradigm on its own is insufficient to administer effective health care for the terminally-ill. Thus, I will argue that it is necessary to extend and supplement the physician-centered paradigm to include the patient's personal and medical needs which must be defined by the patient him/herself. It, therefore, follows that humane health care presupposes that an equal partnership is developed between physician and patient. This will give the patient the necessary psychological support when making end-of-life decisions.

I. Features of the Physician-Patient Relationship

The physician-centered approach is central to the diagnostic method for treating the terminally ill. According to this approach, the physician does not merely diagnose the illness and disclose the alternative treatments which are available to the patient, but (s)he should decide what the patient should do without consulting the patient. Thus, the physician is viewed as an expert and an authority figure for the patient. Since the physician has the medical expertise to cure the patient or at least ease his/her pain and suffering, (s)he has the power to influence the patient to accept whatever treatments (s)he prescribes. This approach insists that the patient remain voiceless and vulnerable to the physician's point of view. This approach also undermines a patient's autonomy and dignity since (s)he is not a part of the decision making about the treatment alternatives which are open to him/her.

There are two main types of physician-patient relationship: (1) the physician-centered relationship; and (2) the patient-centered relationship. I will devote this chapter to the physician -centered approach. In the process, I will also point out some of the difficulties with this paternalistic approach of caring for the terminally ill. According to the physician-centered approach, the patient's position is one of vulnerability and compromised autonomy because of the power differential between physician and patients. The physician-centered approach holds that no amount of patient empowerment can eradicate these vulnerabilities and inherent inequalities. I beg to differ on this point. As I will argue later, most of these inequalities can be remedied if the patient and physician can be viewed as equal partners with the common goal of improving overall health. The alternative approach presupposes that a patient should be respected because (s)he is an autonomous agent who can and must be encouraged to make medical decisions which cohere with his/her values, beliefs, life plans and overall medical goals. No physician can respect patient autonomy without allowing and even encouraging patients to make such decisions for themselves. I will say more about this later.

There are five defining features of the physician-centered approach. First, according to this approach, there is a marked difference in knowledge between physician and patient. The physician has an immense amount of medical knowledge that the patient does not have or even understand in some cases. Thus, the physician knows more about the illness and treatment than the patient. Having such limited information about his/her illness, the patient is unable to make an informed decision about the best medical intervention for him/herself. This makes the patient inept at making his/her own medical decision without the physician's input. Thus, a type of paternalism becomes necessary in order for the patient to agree with the physician's diagnosis, prognosis, and medical treatment. Much of the decision-making power must remain with the physician.

Second, according to this model, the physician must decide what information and how much should be given to the patient in need of treatment. In other words, according to this model, the physician has the ultimate power to decide what should be communicated to the patient. The patient's understanding of the nature of the illness, its course, and likely prognosis depends entirely on what the physician chooses to reveal. In other words, how much truth is disclosed to the patient about his ailment is also controlled by the physician. Therefore, the patient is vulnerable to the physician since a patient's understanding regarding treatment is determined by the way the information is presented. Thus, the patient's autonomy is compromised and the open and honest communication that should occur to develop an effective physician-patient relationship is severely compromised. This is especially important for terminally ill patients. Patients need all the medical information available not merely to choose treatment options but also to make plans for their remaining life. Without the disclosure of such information, a patient cannot effectively engage in his/her own future medical planning. A patient cannot make autonomous choices if (s)he is not given a sufficient amount of information on which to base an autonomous decision about a medical intervention.

Thirdly, according to this model, the physician decides which treatment options should be offered to the patient. There is no disclosure or open communication of all the medical alternatives available to the patient. Instead, the physician decides on the patient's behalf what would be the best treatment for the patient. This undermines a patient's autonomy since the physician does not openly and honestly disclose all the treatment options. In addition, the physician does not allow the patient to make an autonomous and informed decision of his/her own. Under this scenario, the physician simply makes a decision for the patient which does not involve the patient. This is especially serious for a terminally-ill patient. There are usually more than one or two options open to a terminally-ill patient. However, open, honest communication is the key in situations in which a patient is terminally-ill.

Fourthly, this model emphasizes the fact that the physicians have the medical skills and knowledge that the patient does not understand. Therefore, the physician cannot fully communicate to the patient about his/her diagnosis, prognosis or treatment options. Although strictly speaking this is true, for the most part, the physician can explain the treatments and diagnosis in terms that the patient could understand by tailoring the information to the individual patient and his/her medical needs. Each patient also has a substantial amount of information about his/her beliefs, values, and long-term goals that the physician lacks and which is essential to personalize the treatment options. Thus, there should be no power differential between physician and patient but instead a power balance. Therefore, the physician-centered model misconstrues a physician's power by restricting a patient's autonomy and undermining his/her beliefs, values, and medical goals. This is an especially important consideration for the terminally-ill patient.

Fifthly, according to this model, the physician is the gatekeeper of resources and has the power to influence the medical care of a particular patient. Although this is true in principle, patients are also gatekeepers of resources that the physician needs. Every patient has a narrative of his/her life and medical situation that is vital for the physician to tailor the medical treatments to the patient. These personal narratives are also resources which the physician needs to administer effective medical care. Lastly, although the physician could influence a patient's medical care, (s)he should refrain from doing so since it undermines a patient's autonomy and sense of trust. Instead, the physician should strive to openly and honestly discuss a patient's diagnosis, prognosis and treatment. The way the physician discloses the medical information should be unbiased and uninfluenced by a physician's personal agenda. This is especially important when treating the terminally-ill. The physician must refrain from framing the outcome of a treatment in terms of a patient's pending death.

Thus, there are many difficulties to a strictly physician-centered approach to medicine, and this is especially the case when treating the terminally-ill. As will become apparent subsequently, the physician and patient must be equal partners in the terminally-ill patient's care. It is never appropriate for a physician to make a medical decision on the patient's behalf, unless the patient is in a coma or senile. If the patient is unable to make an immediate decision for him/herself, the physician must either consult a patient's advance directives which would have been prepared by the patient ahead of time or contact the patient's trustee, who was appointed by the patient to serve his/her best interest when (s)he is no longer able to do so him/herself. However, at no point can the physician decide what a patient should do in a given medical situation. At most, the physician should merely offer advice to the patient or trustee.

II. Difficulties with the Physician-Centered Paradigm

In this section, I will outline seven key difficulties with a strictly physician-centered paradigm. First, when the medical encounter is physician-centered the communication between patient and physician is one-sided since the physician controls the discussion by prescribing that the patient undergo a particular treatment. There is no necessity for the physician to disclose all the alternative treatments. Within the physician-centered approach, the physician does not merely refrain from disclosing the alternative treatments which are available to the patient, but the physician also decides which treatment would most benefit the patient. But how does the physician know the best treatment without consulting with the patient and openly and honestly discussing the patient's values and desires in relation to the illness and the treatment options available to the particular patient? Throughout the book, I will argue that an open and honest communication with the patient about the diagnosis, prognosis and future treatment options is necessary in order to administer effective health care.

This is especially the case for terminally-ill patients. Patient trust is significantly undermined, if not destroyed completely, if a physician simply tells a patient that there are no viable treatments available to the patient, given his/her illness without initially communicating at length with the patient about some of the possible options. The physician should strive to communicate with the patient about his/her options without maligning the decision with his/her own. A terminally-ill patient already feels vulnerable and out of control because of his/her illness. When a physician determines a patient's medical outcome, the patient is further disrespected and (s)he may feela total lack of control. Humanistic medicine presupposes that the patient must be included in all medical decision-making, especially those decisions which are made at the end of life.

Second, the relationship between the patient and physician is too one-sided for mutual trust and respect to be effectively developed and fostered. The physician centered approach presumes that the physician is an authority figure and is in charge of determining the treatment alternatives for a particular patient. The patient is presumed to be incapable of making medical decisions about treatments because (s)he lacks the medical expertise to make such decisions. Although this is true in part, it does not present the whole story since the patient's beliefs, values and life plans must also enter into whatever future treatments are best for him/her. Say a terminally ill patient really wants to finish writing a novel or run his/her last ten kilometer race before fully giving in to his illness. Within the physician-centered approach, the physician need not discuss a patient's future plans, beliefs, and desires but simply needs to prescribe the treatment (s)he believes will be best for the patient. In many cases, the physician would hamper an important goal that a patient wants to fulfill before (s)he passes away. This undermines a patient's autonomy and shows a disrespect for the patient.

In order to develop mutual trust and respect, the physician and patient must develop an inclusive two-sided relationship. This presupposes that to develop trust, the patient's narrative must enter essentially into the patient's experience of illness and his/her future plans. For instance, if the terminally-ill patient wants to run a ten kilometer race in a few months, the physician should have taken this into consideration when determining what the best treatment option is for a particular patient, given his/her future aspirations. A physician should not assume that all patients have no future aspirations if they become terminally ill.[1] Some patients might still have goals and aspirations that they may want to engage in, despite their terminal illness.[2] Ideally, a terminally-ill patient should be encouraged to do as much as (s)he wants, given his/her medical situation, and its terminality. The physician-centered paradigm misses this important part of a patient's reality when determining the best medical treatment.

Third, the physician-centered model focuses on an impossible power differential between physician and patient, hindering the development of an effective and humane relationship. In fact, the supposed power differential between physician and patient stifles any possibility for developing an open, honest relationship. If a physician believes and acts as if (s)he is superior, the patient will inadvertently be regarded as inferior because of his/her lack of medical knowledge. Once a physician believes that patient is inferior, (s)he will talk down to him/her and refrain from discussing any of the important features of his/her illness on the assumption that (s)he will not understand anyway so why bother. This attitude undermines a patient's autonomy and is disrespectful towards the patient and his/her medical predicament both now and in the future.

This attitude of superiority and inferiority can also bias the physician's attitude towards the patient. In order for humane medicine to occur, the physician must develop a physician and patient relationship that is based on equality and partnership. This presupposes that the physician must allow the patient to make medical decisions in collaboration with the physician. The patient must express his/her overall goals and future life plans with the physician before an appropriate medical treatment can be suggested. Otherwise, the treatment will be suited to the illness but not to the patient who is experiencing the illness. This approach undermines the patient as an individual since it disrespects his/her autonomy and fails to treat the patient as a unique individual who has an illness which will claim this particular individual's life. Thus, the physician-centered approach is quite deficient in achieving this type of humane and inclusive health care.

Fourth, an open and honest physician-patient relationship cannot be developed when the physician simply prescribes the treatment options without the patient's consent. A physician must spend some time discussing the treatment alternatives with the patient. The physician must strive to engage the patient in any of the initial decision making about his/her future health. An open and honest physician-patient relationship can only be developed when the physician openly discloses the patient's diagnosis, prognosis, and future health plan. The physician must also develop a rapport and connection with the patient that goes beyond words. The physician and patient must feel comfortable about discussing anything with one another that pertains to a patient's health. The patient must also feel able to broach any topic whatsoever with the physician. This is especially necessary if a patient is terminally-ill. The development of such an open and honest communication is impossible to achieve on the physician-centered approach.

Fifth, trust is usually undermined and badly hampered within a strictly physician-centered approach since there is an insufficient amount of interaction between physician and patient for trust to be fostered and developed. A patient may say that (s)he trusts his/her physician to prescribe what is best for his/her ailment. However, apparent blind trust is not the kind of trust that is necessary for humane medicine. It is not necessary for a patient to relinquish all consent in order to show that (s)he trusts his/her physician. Instead, trust must be developed, not merely assumed. To develop trust, the physician must include the patient in all aspects of the medical decisions that are relevant to the patient's overall health. This is especially the case for a terminally-ill patient who must openly and honestly communicate with his/her physician to achieve a state of psychological and physical comfort. This cannot be achieved with a strictly physician-centered approach since the trust between physician and patient is merely implied and does not lead to an open honest relationship.

Sixth, in the physician-centered approach, a patient fails to properly consent to treatment that will be administered since to merely agree with the treatment that the physician prescribes is not to consent to it in an informed manner. In the medical setting, to agree usually means to unreflectively and passively go along with whatever the physician prescribes without asking for more information or any clarification. To agree also means to place all the control and decision-making power in the physician's hands. In other words, when a patient ureflectively agrees, (s)he relinquishes all control and wants the physician to paternalistically take care of all his/her health needs without the necessity of consultation. For the purposes of humane medicine and according to the patient-centered approach consent must be informed in order for it to be considered proper consent. For truly informed consent, the patient must understand the diagnosis and the treatments available, along with the risks and benefits of each treatment. Only with this information can the patient give an informed consent about which treatment (s)he prefers.

This is especially important in the case of a terminally ill patient. Many times, after a negative diagnosis is given, such a patient may not be able to effectively process any of the information about the treatments that are available to him/her. This is usually because a negative diagnosis may cause the patient (and even the physician) to bias all treatments in terms of that negative diagnosis. This may further cause the patient to make an irrational decision about what treatments are best for that patient, given his/her medical condition. Thus, it may be better for the physician to schedule two appointments, one for the diagnosis and one for discussing the treatments. Nevertheless, it is absolutely necessary that the patient gives a properly informed and autonomous consent for a medical treatment since, without this, consent becomes mere agreement which violates the patient's autonomy.

Seventh, abuses are more likely to occur if a physician merely sets out to prescribe and administer a patient's treatment without his/her consent. Without discussing the medical alternatives that are available, the patient is left out of the decision-making process. In addition, without open and honest communication, a physician is unaware of the patient's beliefs, values and life plans. This doubly undermines a patient's autonomy and keeps a patient subservient to his/her physician. In addition, the physician, not knowing the patient's true intentions, may become irrationally influenced by a family member or relative who seems to know a patient's best interests yet in actuality fail to.

Conclusion

Given these difficulties with the physician-centered model, it is essential to supplement it with a patient-centered approach which focuses on preserving a patient's autonomy in order to develop a humanistic approach to medicine. What is missing in a strictly physician-centered approach is the patient and his/her narrative of illness. Without forming a partnership, a genuine physician-patient relationship, the physician cannot correctly determine the patient's best treatment options on his/her own. This is especially the case with end-of-life issues since a patient's beliefs, values, and life plans must enter essentially into any future treatment plans that the patient will decide on in collaboration with the physician. At no point should a physician decide what a patient should do in a given terminal situation on his/her own without openly and honestly discussing the alternatives of treatment that are available with the patient in detail. Otherwise, the physician will be undermining a patient's autonomy.

Chapter 4

The Patient-Centered Approach

The term 'patient-centered medicine' was introduced over thirty years ago by Balint (1970) et al[1] who contrasted it with 'illness-centered medicine'. An understanding of the patient's medical concerns that were based on patient-centered thinking was referred to as 'overall diagnosis' while an apprehension of the patient's concerns based on disease-centered thinking was called a "traditional diagnosis". The former was referred to as the patient-centered clinical method while the latter was the doctor-centered approach.[2] The doctor-centered approach has been and still is extremely seductive in medical practice; however, it must be supplemented or replaced with the patient-centered approach in order for the "whole patient" to be taken into consideration.[3] This is especially important when patients become terminally-ill and must make difficult decisions about medical interventions and treatment plans.

Disease is a theoretical construct through which physicians can explain a patient's medical concerns in terms of the abnormalities of a patient's bodily organs. Illness refers to a patient's personal experience of disease since illness is unique for each patient.[4] For instance, stomach cancer will be experienced differently by each patient despite the fact that the symptoms are similar. A patient-centered approach requires that the physicians attend carefully to a patient's personal experience of illness as well as the symptoms of his/her disease. To identify a patient's disease solely on the basis of certain bodily abnormalities is common to the conventional medical approach, while understanding the patient's experience of illness presupposes an additional focus. A patient-centered approach focuses on the disease and at least four additional dimensions of a patient's experience of illness, such as his/her ideas about what is wrong with him, his/her feelings and fears about the illness, the impact of his/her medical problems on proper bodily function, and his/her expectations about what should be done to ameliorate the medical situation.

Thus, the central features of this approach are the physical and psychological cues related to these dimensions.[5] The goal of the patient-centered approach is for a physician to understand a patient's experience of illness from that patient's perspective. In order to achieve a therapeutic understanding of the patient's experience of illness, a physician must develop interpersonal skills to enable him/her to 'enter into the patient's world' and to understand a patient's illness from that patient's unique point of view. Thus, the physician must become empathic with a patient's medical predicament. Some patients will be better at expressing their experience of illness than others. However, most patients will find it difficult to clearly communicate their feelings about their illness. So, the physician may have to ask open ended questions such as "How does having such a pain or discomfort affect you?" and then give the patient a sufficient amount of time to respond. Response times will vary from patient to patient as a result of differences in character, beliefs, values and life experiences. The physician must leave an ample amount of time for the patient to respond. It is helpful for the physician to get to know a patient's background by extensively talking to him/her over time, preferably before (s)he becomes terminally ill.

Thus, the physician must strive to understand the patient as a whole person before and during the onset of the illness. This requires that the physician gather a sufficient amount of medical, and especially personal, information about the patient that goes beyond diagnosing disease or attending to the biological responses of illness. In the process, the physician will start understanding the patient's experience of illness in the context of his/her life. The knowledge that the physician acquires about the patient may include information about the family, work, and struggles with various life crises. The physician who understands the patient as a whole person recognizes the impact of the family in ameliorating, aggravating or even causing illness in its members. The patient's cultural beliefs and attitudes can also influence the medical care (s)he prefers. Thus, an understanding of the whole patient can also enhance personal and interpersonal communication with patients. Understanding the patient in this complete way underlies the patient-centered approach and the four conditions outlined below. The traditional clinical method fails to focus on the patient's unique experience of illness, and is thus deficient in developing humane health care for a terminally ill patient.

I. Rebuilding The Traditional Clinical Method

Some theorists may ask: Why do we need a new clinical method when the traditional paradigm seems good enough? One answer to the question could be divided into two distinct parts. First, although the traditional paradigm of medicine may be acceptable to most physicians, this is not the case for the patient since within the doctor-centered approach, physicians and patients have different goals for medicine. Second, the traditional paradigm of medicine undermines the patient's autonomy, making him feel more vulnerable and less in control of his/her health. This can have tragic consequences for the terminally ill patient. Even from a medical perspective, our present therapeutic method is failing to meet the needs of the twentieth century. Our diagnostic and therapeutic methods, the structure of the medical profession, and the health care system are mostly products of the enlightenment.[6] No wonder the therapeutic method is unable to deal with the medical issues that are unique to the technologically driven twentieth century.

Our first task in rebuilding the clinical method is to recapture the capacity to respond to the patient reflectively and spontaneously. A patient prefers to be recognized, appreciated, and understood.[7] This means that a physician must appropriately respond to a patient's suffering. One of medicine's perennial moral problems is a failure to respond to suffering. Truly caring for a patient has very little, if anything, to do with categories: instead, caring shows the patient that his/her life is valuable because it recognizes the uniqueness of his/her experience of illness.[8] A physician should respond to a patient's suffering by being empathically moved by his/her whole being. Thus, the goals of medicine must change from merely focusing on a diagnosis and prognosis to appreciating the nature of a patient's illness and how the patient is affected by it.

One of the most important ways that a physician could recognize a patient's suffering is by carefully listening to the patient's narrative of illness with undivided attention. This could be achieved by sitting at the patient's bedside, attending to the physical and psychological needs to ensure that (s)he is comfortable, and being present at a critical time when a patient needs support by asking a question that may release pent-up emotions and feelings. These patients will feel more cared for and less vulnerable. These acts are also beneficial for the physician to appreciate the patient's genuine medical predicament and how (s)he is feeling as a result of the illness. Terminal illness can affect not only a patient's physical health but his/her overall psychological makeup by biasing future treatments as ways of prolonging pain and suffering. The physician must try as much as possible to dissuade the patient from irrationally biasing his/her interpretations of future treatments in this way.

Lastly, the physician must determine what impact the terminal illness will have on the patient's life by considering the limitations, disabilities, effects on relationships, work, interests, hopes, and future aspirations. This information can be beneficial for a physician in determining the amount of care that is necessary for a terminally-ill patient to feel as comfortable and in control as possible. A physician must also become aware of the patient's understanding of his/her illness, such as his/her sense of what caused the disease, the patient's expectations of the doctor, the patient's feelings and emotions towards his/her illness, and his/her expectations about the illness. This understanding will lead the physician and patient to a common ground, and especially a mutual understanding about the patient's experience of illness affected by it.

The most difficult change that is necessary to transform the clinical method is the transition from linear, causal thinking about disease to a cybernetic and global way. Linear thinking is unidirectional from cause to effect. The notion of 'cybernetic causation' is based on the model of self-organizing systems. A human being can be viewed as a self-organizing system, maintaining itself by interaction with its environment and by a system of feedback loops from the environment and from its own inner output loops. Typically, self-organizing systems are not as passive as linear ones since they have the ability to renew and transcend themselves. However, self-organizing systems require energy to maintain. In self-organizing systems, the notion of cause is based on the model of information which triggers a process of self-discernment. In the clinical encounter, physicians must consider the processes in the organism that are perpetuating a physical and psychological disturbance in the patient. The key to enhancing a patient's process of psychological healing is to strengthen his/her defences and encourage self-transcendence, rather than neutralizing the patient.

II. The Changing Scene of Medicine

Four revisions have contributed to the changing paradigm of medicine. First, there has been an increased emphasis on patient autonomy. It is no longer sufficient for the physician to merely treat the patient's disease but (s)he must also include the whole person who has the disease. When a patient becomes seriously ill, his/her whole person is affected. In addition, often the patient's personal history and life have had a major impact on the development of the disease. All of this is part of the disease and must be taken into consideration in order to respect a patient's autonomy at the time of diagnosis and prognosis. I will say much more about this in Part II of the book.

Second, the biomolecular revolution and other new technologies in medicine have substantially improved and changed the texture of patient-care. Medical care can be administered twenty four hours a day, seven days a week. The introduction of technologies that permit rapid diagnosis by CAT scanning and magnetic imaging, the development of interventional radiology and angiography, and the capacity to treat cardiac arrhythmias and heart failure with new drugs and sophisticated devices have radically changed the nature of hospital care.[9] This has had serious consequences for the physician-patient relationship. Physicians and staff merely pass each other without necessarily talking to one another. They generally have no time to pause for a minute.

In addition, numbers have become the most important measuring aspect for most physicians since, for instance, the number given to the patient's chest pain often overshadows some of the other terms which describe the quality of pain. Many times, chest pain is described in numerical terms so that if a patient has had repeated visits to the emergency room, they often came in complaining of "8 out of 10 chest pain".[10] This is sad statement of how the new technology has affected patient care. It seems that quantitative information is judged to be more important, reliable, and valid than qualitative and narrative data in arriving at medical decisions. This makes the patient's narrative less important in medicine, which reduces the importance for physicians to administer Humane medicine. Although the new diagnostic tests greatly enhance the physician's ability to diagnose a patient's illness accurately and treat it effectively, they cannot fully address the unique aspects of illness that bring the patient and physician into a relationship whose importance is not diminished even as medicine becomes increasingly scientific. It is essential for physicians to understand the numbers while retaining their sensitivity to the unique aspects of illness in this era of the Biomedical Revolution.[11] I will say more about this in Part III.

Third, there has been an increased emphasis on informed consent in medicine the main purpose of which is for physicians to avoid malpractice lawsuits. A secondary reason for ensuring that a patient gives an informed consent for a medical procedure is to include the patient in the decision-making process. According to the biomolecular revolution, the reason for including the patient is not necessarily to respect a patient's autonomy but to protect the physician. I believe that this view fails to capture the essence of the patient-centered approach since respecting a patient's autonomy should be given top priority. Anyhow, in the process, the physician will also be protecting him/herself from legal ramifications. It is essential that the patient become of central importance in the medical interaction, given the biomolecular revolution and its emphasis on the scientific aspect of medicine.

Fourth, there is increased attention given to prevention and patient education. Patients are now able to research medical information on the internet. Much of this process has been due to the biomolecular revolution. Patients can become aware of what they can do to reduce the risk of heart disease, cancer, diabetes and so on. This is important information for the conscientious patient who feels motivated to stay as healthy as possible for as long as possible. However, given the carcinogens in our environment, patients must also avoid being exposed to these cancer-causing agents, if possible. Thus, the emphasis on prevention and education does ensure that the patient can control his/her health more readily, by working closely with the physician.

However, there are five strains which affect achieving humane health care, given the biomolecular revolution. First, the rapid changes in medicine have caused a dichotomy or tension to develop between an emphasis on ensuring that a patient's autonomy is respected and the medical profession's insistence that diagnostic techniques continue to improve. This can also create gaps in the process of developing a patient-centered approach to medicine. Let me dwell a bit more on the tension that is at stake. The new paradigm has emphasized that the science of medicine is most important since drastic improvements have been made to diagnostic and preventative techniques because of it. The consequences to the new paradigm is that although there is an emphasis on informed consent and patient-autonomy, the patient's qualitative, experiential aspects of illness have been eliminated. Thus, according to the new paradigm, the respect for the patient that is advocated does not benefit the patient as much as the medical profession.

In other words, although physicians are aware that some of their patients are capable and knowledgeable enough to make decisions about their health, the new diagnostic techniques which are part of the biomolecular revolution are reducing patients to numbers and creating even a further distance between physicians and patients. Thus, physicians do not have the time or inclination to discuss the patient's experience of illness. The quantitative methodology for describing pain is quickly catching on. A few days ago, I asked a friend of mine, how she was feeling and she said "Oh, about forty out of fifty." I found that description to be alarming since she always used to say either "Today, I feel a lot of pain" or "Today, I feel very little pain." When I asked her why she changed the way she described her pain level she said "My doctor wants me to get into the habit of describing pain quantitatively. I found it hard at first, but now I think that I am catching on all right". Obviously, Elizabeth's physician wants to familiarize her with a qualitative analysis of pain so that the qualitative and experiential features of the illness are no longer relevant to their future discussion. This is cumbersome because most patients can only describe illness in qualitative terms.

The second difficulty caused by the biomolecular revolution is that the physician must ensure that his/her patient always gives an informed consent for a medical procedure. But who is the physician trying to protect? Given the stress of the new biomolecular paradigm of medicine on the quantitative aspects of illness, it seems that physicians are trying to protect themselves instead of the patient. Once the forms are signed, the physician is not liable for any damages which occur. While originally the aim of obtaining an informed consent was for the patient's autonomy to be respected, currently, the patient's autonomy seems to be of secondary importance. Physicians believe that they should protect themselves against all legal ramifications first. This way of viewing informed consent is wrong headed since a patient's autonomy is still violated.

Instead, I will argue that the patient should be protected first and foremost when a physician gets an informed consent. When the patient is respected and given a choice of medical treatments, the physician will also be protected since the patient will be comfortable with the diagnosis and prognosis of his/her illness. This respect and care will help the patient feel much more comfortable and less likely to complain about the physician's behavior or actions. Thus, by respecting a patient's autonomy and ensuring that the main purpose of an informed consent is to protect the patient, the physician can ensure that patient-centered health care is administered. Given the new paradigm of medicine, this is of utmost importance to achieve, especially for a terminally-ill patient.

Third, advocates of the biomolecular revolution believe that it has greatly benefited health care and the prevention of disease. Although this is correct in part, the biomolecular revolution has also had some serious consequences for patient care. First, the patient's illness and experience of illness has been dehumanized substantially because of the physician's emphasis on the quantitative aspects of illness instead of the qualitative and experiential features. The quantitative descriptions of illness have reduced feelings and emotions of illness to a numerical code. Most patients find it difficult to quantitatively describe their pain levels, while they feel more comfortable discussing how their pain curtailed their daily activities or made sleeping or eating difficult.

The fourth difficulty with the new biomolecular revolution is that an open and honest physician-patient relationship cannot be fostered or developed effectively. The new paradigm only insists that the physician have a formal discussion with a patient about his/her illness. The personal and experiential features of the illness are missing. Every patient has a name and a story of his/her illness which must be listened to attentively and discussed openly and honestly with the physician. The challenge for the physician is to develop the skills and sensitivity to really listen to the patient's story and then to discuss the patient's medical options and diagnosis openly and honestly. The more a physician communicates with the patient, the more likely it will be that (s)he will develop an open, honest and trusting relationship with that patient. This may also ensure that the physician will have a more nurturing and enjoyable relationship with the patient which will enrich his/her experience as a doctor.[12]

The fifth difficulty is that the new biomolecular revolution tends to be paternalistic. Since a physician insists on quantifying the experience of illness, the patient feels unable to comprehend the physician's explanations. This creates a gap in the patient's ability to contribute to medical decisions about his/her illness. Thus, patients feel left out and their autonomy is undermined when they cannot understand and fully communicate with the physician. Shared decision-making becomes an impossible obstacle for most patients. Within the patient-centered approach to medicine, this cannot be permitted. The patient must be encouraged to make decisions about his/her health care with the physician. It is essential in the patient-centered approach for a physician to ensure that a patient contributes to shared decision-making for a medical intervention.

III. Reconciling The New Biomolecular Revolution

The patient-centered approach is not antithetical to the new biomolecular paradigm and the two facets of medicine could be reconciled to form a complete account for palliative care and the terminally-ill patient since there are no necessary tensions between the new paradigm and the patient-centered approach. All that is needed to reconcile the two facets of medicine is for the patient to enter more prominently into the medical encounter. This means that along with the emphasis on charts and numbers, the physician should also focus on the patient's experience of illness. In this way, the patient can reap the benefits and advances from the new paradigm and still have personalized health care. A terminally-ill patient needs the most advanced medical techniques in order to achieve the best quality of life until death. In addition, a physician needs to administer the most effective pain medication to the terminally-ill patient. In this way, the patient will feel genuinely taken care of and comforted. This presupposes that the physician is empathic and focuses on how the illness is affecting the patient.

Thus, to provide a blending of the new molecular paradigm of medicine with the patient-centered approach, the physician should engage in a qualitative and quantitative assessment of the illness. The qualitative assessment would involve the personal aspects of the terminal illness, such as the patient's beliefs, values, goals, career plans, and expectations while the quantitative assessment will involve the scientific and biomolecular technologies that are part of the new paradigm of medicine. Terminally-ill patients deserve to have the most up-to-date treatments administered to help alleviate some of their symptoms. I believe that terminally-ill patients need both the patient-centered, personal approach and the new paradigm of medicine.This will ensure that the terminally-ill patient receives the best medical care which is personalized to his/her medical and psychological needs.

Conclusion

In Part II, I will discuss in more detail the five features of the patient-centered approach to medicine and I will leave it to each physician to integrate the approach developed into the new biomolecular model. There is no need to argue that the new paradigm of medicine reaffirms the traditional, paternalistic doctor-centered approach. I believe that the biomolecular revolution is absolutely crucial to effective health care for terminally ill patients in the new millennium. However, I also believe that physicians cannot afford to simply focus on the medical improvements of medicine without giving some attention to the interpersonal features of terminal illness. The terminally-ill patient requires both the best types of medical care combined with humane health care so that (s)he can feel cared for and comfortable.

Chapter 5

Effective Physician-Patient Disclosure

The purpose of this chapter is to discuss the importance of effective communication between the physician and patient in this new biomolecular millennium of medicine for the terminally-ill. There are four main dimensions of an effective disclosure: (1) open and honest discussion; (2) understanding between physician and patient; (3) discussion of the psychological influences of diagnosis; and (4) being empathic with and sensitive to a patient's situation. Each of these dimensions of disclosure will be beneficial in helping the terminally-ill patient to more readily accept his/her illness. These dimensions can also help the patient get over the initial shock and grief of the negative diagnosis news.

In this chapter, I will examine each of these dimensions with the intention of developing a humane, patient-centered approach that is especially applicable for the terminally-ill patient when (s)he must make a decision about a treatment. Effective disclosure is very difficult to achieve, especially for a patient who has just learned that (s)he has a terminal disease. Initially, the patient is usually grief-stricken and can become depressed and silent, refraining from talking to anyone due to fear. Eventually, the fear turns to anger, and at this point the physician may discover that it is very difficult, it not impossible, to communicate with the patient. Thus, ideally it is best for the physician to build a relationship of mutual trust and respect before the patient becomes terminally ill. However, should this not be possible, the physician must strive to develop effective disclosure as soon as the patient is diagnosed with a terminal illness.

I. Open, Honest Discussion and Disclosure

When the physician discovers that his/her patient has a terminal illness, (s)he must disclose the diagnosis as openly and honestly as possible. There are some physicians who may feel initially shocked and grief stricken themselves that a particular patient is terminally-ill. If this is the case, the physician may find it easier to take a day or two to come to terms with news of the patient's illness and then set up an appointment to discuss the diagnosis with the patient. It is not inappropriate for a physician to take some time to 'digest' the diagnosis. This is especially the case if the physician has been caring for the patient for some time. If the physician takes the time (s)he feels that is needed, (s)he will be better able to help the patient deal with the initial shock of the negative news and then ensure that the patient does not lose hope but is able to cope with the diagnosis and prognosis. This is why the physician must remain 'open' to the patient's psychological concerns about his/her illness. The patient must never feel pressured to disclose feelings (s)he is not ready to express or be made to feel that (s)he is wasting a physician's time. Thus, the physician should usually schedule at least a one hour time slot to discuss the diagnosis, and to give the patient a sufficient amount of time to express sadness, fears, anxieties, or to ask whatever questions come to mind.

There are two central aspects of effective disclosure, and this is especially so when the physician is disclosing the negative news to the patient for the first time. First, openness and honesty is necessary as the physician discloses the diagnosis to the terminally-ill patient. Most theorists categorize 'openness' to be an aspect of honesty. However, the two concepts should be separated in order to be able to clearly distinguish between these two concepts since they have different functions for the purposes of disclosing a terminal diagnosis. 'Openness' typically has a subjective and psychological function in the disclosure while 'honesty' has a much more objective function. When a physician is 'open' to the patient, (s)he should allow him/her to express any emotions or anything which (s)he is perplexed with. In addition, the physician must also express 'openness' through gestures and body language. 'Honesty' usually presupposes that the physician discloses the diagnosis correctly.[1]

The second psychological aspect of openness is that the physician must provide the patient with a sufficient amount of time to respond to the diagnosis, after the initial disclosure. The physician may feel that it is necessary to meet with the patient a few days or a week after the initial disclosure to discuss any other matters and answer any further questions. By then the initial shock usually subsides and the patient should be able to think about his/her future medical treatment plans. The patient must be given as much time as is necessary to allow him/her to come to terms with an illness. Each terminally ill patient will have a unique ability to cope with the shock of the diagnosis. Thus, the physician must determine how much time is necessary for each patient.

The first physical component of 'openness' is the necessity for the physician to sit within arm's reach of the patient when disclosing the negative diagnosis so as to be able to comfort him/her if it is necessary. This closeness usually signifies a sense of emotional openness to the patient. Second, the physician must gesture freely and speak in a low, comforting voice which expresses concern. The physician may also use empathic and reassuring language when discussing the diagnosis such as:

> "I know this must be shocking to you."
> "I know how devastating this news must be to you."
> "I'm sure you were not expecting to hear this."
> "I know how hard it must be for you to hear such a diagnosis."

The physician may also feel that it is appropriate to ask the patient how (s)he is feeling and whether there is any way (s)he could help the patient. The physician may suggest that the patient speak with a nurse practitioner or a counselor. The patient should always be given many different opportunities to discuss his/her feelings and emotions. Lastly, the physician should use reassuring statements such as: "I will make sure that you are cared for until the end."

'Honesty' also has an objective component in the diagnosis and prognosis.[2] The physician must disclose the results of the patient's diagnosis in detail without holding any aspect of it back. If the tests come back inconclusive, that should also be disclosed. For instance, after running a few x-rays, the physician may discover that the patient has a tumor on the top of the right lung. Most times, tumors on the lung are cancerous; however, a small percentage are nonmalignant. The patient should be informed of all of the uncertainties that are inherent in the test results. Thus, it is inappropriate for the physician to withhold any aspect of the test results. In addition, in some cases, it may be appropriate to disclose the diagnosis over several meetings. This is especially the case if the patient does not understand English fluently or is emotional and cannot effectively process a negative diagnosis.

II. Effective Understanding

An effective disclosure of a diagnosis presupposes that the patient understands the diagnosis, prognosis and treatment alternatives disclosed by the physician. Generally, an effective disclosure is characterized as an exchange between two individuals that has the overriding purpose of giving information and assisting understanding.[3] Understanding may be characterized as the patient's assimilation of the information about the medical alternatives of treatment disclosed by the physician. The criteria for understanding the disclosure of the diagnosis is complex since it involves psychological and intellectual idiosyncrasies which are unique to each patient. Each patient's degree and level of understanding must be intuitively assessed by the physician in order to determine how much information a particular patient can absorb about the alternative treatments and procedures and whether the terminally ill patient will require special considerations, such as a reiteration of the diagnosis.

Several factors may be instrumental in ensuring that a disclosure is properly understood by the patient.

According to the patient-centered model developed in this work, a terminally ill patient must substantially understand the diagnosis, prognosis and disclosure about the treatments. A substantial amount of information must be disclosed by the physician about the possible treatment alternatives which are available to the patient. Some of the types of medical information that must be disclosed include:

(1)	the diagnosis;
(2)	all the risks and benefits which are involved in each medical alternative;
(3)	the success rate of each procedure based on past records;
(4)	the pain level that can be expected for each treatment alternative;
(5)	an estimation of recuperation time; and
(6)	a detailed description and ranking of each treatment.

Each of these factors requires a relatively detailed disclosure by the physician and a certain amount of time to process the information by the patient. This is especially so for the last factor of disclosure since assessment requires a ranking of the alternative treatments. This presupposes that the patient has understood all the medical alternatives. Understanding this information is a complex process, and this is especially the case for a terminally ill patient. The more carefully and empathically a physician explicates the treatment alternatives, the more completely a patient will understand the information disclosed.

There are three conditions for understanding the diagnosis. These are:

1.	Shared understanding;
2.	Determining the relevancy of information disclosed; and
3.	Using medical jargon sparingly.[4]

(1) Shared understanding occurs when the physician understands the details of the patient's values, goals, beliefs, and life plans. In addition, the patient must understand that the physician operates within certain medical constraints which are, in effect, beyond his/her control as well. Both the physician and patient must comprehend each other in a subjective, person-to-person manner, which allows each of them to openly and honestly communicate without manipulation or possible disingenuousness. The terminally-ill patient's feelings of grief and vulnerability can be greatly eased with a shared understanding of that patient's predicament.

There is an important distinction between "shared understanding" and "ordinary understanding". Shared understanding is based on a reciprocal understanding between patient and physician, and this is a central feature of a patient's understanding of the medical alternatives. Ordinary understanding consists of the physician merely communicating the facts of the treatment alternatives available to the patient, and risks and benefits without attempting to take the patient's personal needs and values into consideration. It is insufficient for the physician to simply communicate the raw facts of the alternative treatments and the risks and benefits to the patient since the physician must "personalize" the treatment alternatives to the particular terminally ill patient based on his/her personal values, goals, beliefs and life plans. These personal features of the treatment alternatives must be determined through effective communication and a "shared" understanding between physician and patient.

(2) Initially, the physician must disclose all the alternative treatments available, without prioritizing them. Then the patient and physician must eliminate the irrelevant treatment alternatives together, evaluating the remaining alternatives in greater detail. It should never merely be the physician's responsibility to decide which treatment alternatives are relevant to a particular terminally ill patient. Relevancy is difficult to determine because it is usually unique to the emotional state of the patient. The personal and psychological aspects of a terminally ill patient are difficult to unravel without communicating with the patient at length. Ensuring that a terminally ill patient is included in the process of choosing the relevant alternatives of treatment invites him/her into the decision-making process for his/her own terminal illness. This, in turn, ensures that the patient feels more secure, less vulnerable, and more in control of the final stages of his/her disease. This kind of shared decision making also ensures that the patient is competent to decide what treatment alternative s(he) will undergo, which usually results in faster recovery for patients.

(3) If the treatment alternatives are disclosed to the patient in a technical manner, (s)he will probably not be able to fully understand the disclosure. The physician should be aware that the patient is immersed in medical jargon that has taken the doctor many years to master. Medical jargon becomes second nature to the physician; thus, s(he) may unintentionally disclose the medical alternatives in a technical manner. Physicians should remember that medical terminology is usually considered to be a convenient short-hand; but it can and should be translated into ordinary language so that the patient is able to understand. The patient has no medical training, and although patients are better informed about health matters today than a few decades ago, technical jargon can still make it impossible for most patients to understand the disclosure. Thus, the physician should be extremely careful about how much medical language (s)he uses when disclosing information about the alternative treatments available to a terminally ill patient.

An understanding of the alternative treatments is especially difficult to achieve for some terminally ill patients. The degree of the difficulty in achieving an effective understanding depends on many factors, such as:

(1) Levels of education;
(2) Capacities for reflectiveness; and
(3) Psychological factors such as: (i) initial shock of diagnosis; (ii) relentless pain; (iii) feelings of hopelessness and depression; and (iv) grief.

(1) Differing levels of education affect how, or even whether, a terminally ill patient will grasp the medical information disclosed and the amount of time needed to assimilate the information. Terminally ill patients with secondary and

post-secondary education do not pose as serious a problem for physicians as patients who lack secondary education. The latter group of individuals make the practice of understanding the disclosure especially difficult. These difficulties, however, are surmountable. The less education a patient has, the clearer and simpler the information about the medical intervention must be conveyed. However, simplicity must not compromise accuracy or completeness. The physician may also discover that it is necessary to set up additional sessions to explain the treatment alternatives to the terminally ill patient so that (s)he could effectively understand what is disclosed. Patients with lower educational levels may need extra time in order to understand the procedures of the alternative treatments disclosed; however, they must still be able to effectively understand the treatments disclosed if they are to give an informed consent.

(2) Differing levels of patient reflectiveness could also affect a patient's understanding of the alternatives disclosed. It is relatively simple for a physician to determine whether or not a terminally ill patient is sufficiently reflective so that s(he) will not make hasty decisions about medical treatments. Reflective patients: (1) insist on having an adequate amount of time to think about the alternative treatments disclosed, and how each treatment may adversely affect the patient; (2) ask questions about important aspects of treatments that they didn't initially understand; and (3) decide in favor of a given medical treatment on the basis of their values, goals and life plans.

Reflectiveness does not, in principle, depend on the patient's level of education. Most individuals are minimally reflective, although the quality and degree of a patient's reflective capacity may vary substantially. Some patients may be reflective enough to think about the treatment alternatives disclosed by the physician, but may decide to undergo a treatment hastily, not taking the time needed to reflect on the treatment alternatives and their side effects. Such patients usually fail to have a coherent set of values, goals and life plans available for them to make a proper, autonomous choice about a medical treatment. There are also some completely unreflective patients and they pose the most severe difficulties for the physician who is attempting to achieve an informed consent for a medical treatment. The physician must guide an unreflective patient's thinking in an unbiased manner such that s(he) could make a decision which is reflective enough, demonstrating that s(he) has in fact understood the information disclosed by the physician.

(3) Four psychological factors can influence a patient's understanding. These are:

(i)   Initial shock of the diagnosis;
(ii) Relentless pain;
(iii) Feelings of hopelessness and depression; and
(iv) Grief

(i) After the initial shock of the diagnosis, the terminally ill patient may find it difficult to fully understand a physician's disclosure of the disease, much less the treatment alternatives that are available. A terminally ill patient who is in shock initially will not be able to effectively understand and process the information disclosed about the terminal illness. The patient may also become sad or outraged with the diagnosis. To be in shock is to be numb, scared, upset, surprised, in disbelief, dumbfounded, taken aback and uncontrollably sad. It is best in such a situation for the physician to schedule another appointment to disclose the treatment alternatives available to the terminally ill patient since the patient may not be able to digest any more information, given his/her medical distress.

(ii) Relentless pain could also affect a terminally ill patient's capacity for understanding the information about the treatment alternatives available. When a terminally ill patient is in constant pain, s(he) sometimes may experience depression and feelings of vulnerability. The terminally ill patient usually desires to have his/her pain lessened as soon as possible. Such patients may "frame" treatment solutions to their diseases hastily and unreflectively because of their pain and discomfort levels. Physicians, upon recognition of such difficulties, must then guide a terminally ill patient's thinking processes so that (s)he chooses the most appropriate treatment, given his/her values, goals, and deeply held beliefs prior to illness. In this way, the patient may be able to "step back" from his/her pain, or at least reflect on how it was before his/her illness, and make a decision that is based on an understanding of all the treatment alternatives available to him/her.

(iii) Feelings of hopelessness and depression may also be detrimental to a terminally ill patient's capacity for understanding since these can irrationally sway feelings towards inappropriate treatments. The time available for a patient to have a normal and fulfilled life is usually drastically shortened upon discovering that (s)he has a terminal disease. Terminally ill patients will "frame" the treatment alternatives differently from a patient who has an acute illness in which they may be undergoing a routine surgery after which time the patient will recover within a few weeks, resuming his/her normal activities. A terminally ill patient may "frame" his/her decision in a way that is biased towards death, hopelessness and futility. The physician must keep this tendency in mind since the terminally ill patient's decision can sometimes appear irrational and lacking understanding. One possible solution may be for the physician to guide the terminally ill patient's thinking in a way that best reflects the patient's values, goals and life plans prior to his/her illness. This presupposes that the physician has known the terminally ill patient for a substantial time before his/her terminal illness so that the physician is able to tell whether or not a treatment is out of character.

(iv) Grief is a normal process of adapting emotionally to the terminality of a patient's disease. Grief usually disrupts the mental composure of a terminally ill patient for a while. For some terminally ill patients, the grief experienced is stronger and more intense than for others. This could occur for several reasons. First, the terminally ill patient may not have effective coping skills to get through the experience of grief. It may sometimes be necessary for a physician to recommend that the patient see a counselor to cope with the initial shock of the situation. Second, the terminally ill patient may not have a support system in place to express his/her grief in a nurturing environment. The patient may have to develop friendships with other terminally ill patients within a support group for patients with a particular terminal illness. The physician could also help the patient set up such a group. Third, the patient may have never had health problems before and (s)he didn't expect to be terminally ill. Such patients usually are shocked about having a terminal illness. While the experience of grieving is not the same for every patient, there are certain commonalties. During the initial phases, terminally-ill patients should be encouraged to take some time for themselves to recuperate from the initial shock of the negative diagnosis before making important decisions about their health and treatment alternatives.

Unexpressed grief can create many psychological biases in terminally ill patients should they be asked to make decisions about future medical alternatives. For instance, a grief-stricken seventy year old woman who has just learned that (s)he has ovarian cancer may say: "I don't want surgery or chemotherapy. I just want to die naturally." After the initial grief has subsided, the terminally ill patient may be more open to discuss the possibility of surgery and other treatments. Thus, it is essential for physicians to schedule another appointment a few weeks or a month after the initial diagnosis to discuss the treatment alternatives that are available to the patient. Most patients will have difficulty coping with the possibility of imminent death due to their illness because they may be in denial about their pending death.

Thus, a grief-stricken terminally ill patient may have difficulty understanding the information that the physician will disclose. There are several practical tests which a physician could use to determine whether or not a terminally ill patient really understands the information disclosed. First, the physician can ask the terminally ill patient to repeat the information (s)he disclosed in his/her own words. In the process, the physician can determine how much of the information the terminally ill patient has actually understood. Second, the physician may try to disclose the information over several sessions while asking the terminally ill patient after each session to explain the treatment alternative(s) disclosed during that session and/or the previous session (if there was one). After the last session, the terminally ill patient must explain all the treatment alternatives that are available to the physician. This will give the physician a better idea about whether the patient understood the alternatives. The more successfully (i.e., with as few errors as possible) a terminally ill patient explains all the alternatives, the more substantially the patient understands the information disclosed. These explanations serve to reinforce the information for the terminally ill patient so that s(he) does not merely recall them, but will be able to know quite a bit more about the details of the treatment alternatives. This strategy seems to promise a better success rate, owing to the constant reinforcement of the information than the first test, which only stresses that a patient accurately repeat the information after all the disclosure of treatment has been made.

By using these two strategies, physicians can ensure that their patients have understood all the treatments available. This is important because without an understanding of the treatments, patients cannot possibly make an autonomous and rational decision about their treatment, and an informed consent cannot be given. Since physicians have a moral, if not a legal, obligation that patients give an informed consent, they also have a duty to ensure that patients have a substantial understanding of the procedures. The two strategies above could serve as oral tests that the physician could use to determine a patient's capacity for understanding. If the patient fails any of these tests, the physician must repeat the process until the tests are successfully passed.

III. Psychological Discussion of Fears

After the disclosure, the physician must also leave ample amounts of time to discuss a terminally ill patient's fears, both real and imagined. When the physician diagnoses a terminal illness within a patient, (s)he is usually plagued with all kinds of fears. Most times, family members are not available, either physically or psychologically to talk with the patient. Many families do not communicate effectively with each other. This is especially the case when one of the family members becomes seriously ill. Instead, the terminally ill patient usually becomes secretive and refrains from telling the family members the whole truth until (s)he absolutely has to.[5] The terminally ill patient may say that (s)he merely has to undergo some routine tests, and just leave it at that. Only at a much later date, when the terminally patient is weak and visibly sick, will (s)he fully disclose the diagnosis.

Thus, the physician must spend a sufficient amount of time discussing the terminally-ill patient's fears and answering questions such as: "How long do I have to live?", "When will my quality of life start deteriorating?", "How much pain will I have to endure?", "How far has the disease spread?", and so on. These fears will usually plague the patient until (s)he dies. Some of the questions do not have clear-cut answers. There are also imagined fears which the patient should openly discuss with his/her physician. It is essential that the physician discuss these fears as empathically as possible without negatively judging the patient. For instance, the physician may diagnose a patient with lung cancer and presume that (s)he has no more than one year to live. The terminally ill patient may state that (s)he does not want chemotherapy because one of her relatives was so deathly ill after it that her quality of life was substantially reduced. Because of the patient's real and imagined fears, she may simply opt to take pain medication for the remainder of her life and let nature take its course.

Another way the physician could ensure that the terminally ill patient can talk about his/her fears is by asking open-ended questions such as: "How have you felt since the diagnosis?" "Are you scared about the future?" "What scares you the most about your diagnosis?" "What scares you least?" "Can you keep working part-time?" "Which hobbies are most important to you that you can keep doing?" "Do you feel a lot of pain?" "Am I prescribing enough pain medication?" This process is especially important for terminally ill patients who may be having a difficult time discussing their feelings. Most terminally-ill patients will be in shock a long time after a negative diagnosis. When a terminally-ill patient is in shock, (s)he usually becomes silent and sad. By asking open-ended questions, the physician could engage the terminally ill patient and hopefully make it easier for him/her to openly discuss his/her fears.

After a few weeks or months, the physician should also discuss his/her fears about the terminally ill patient. The physician may feel that the terminally ill patient will give up and have a poorer quality of life if (s)he does not at least try chemotherapy. The physician may also feel that the terminally ill patient is not taking care of him/herself sufficiently. Alternatively, the physician may not honestly know precisely how long a terminally ill patient will live, given his/her medical situation. Thus, the physician may fear giving a wrong estimate of time. Telling the terminally ill patient about the uncertainties of the disease can also create an environment for open and honest communication. Further, a physician may also be shocked about a terminally ill patient's diagnosis. Perhaps the terminally ill patient was never seriously ill until diagnosed with a terminal illness. It may be appropriate for the physician to say that (s)he was also shocked with the diagnosis. Such a disclosure can also open lines of communication and help the patient and physician develop a relationship of mutual trust and respect.

IV. Empathic Disclosure

Empathy is another feature of effective disclosure. Many times, the patient may feel insufficiently taken care of because the physician appears to be nonempathic and uncaring. Empathy shows a terminally ill patient that the physician genuinely cares about his/her situation. In empathic listening, a physician should listen with his/her eyes and heart to the terminally ill patient's plea. The physician must also listen for a terminally ill patient's feelings, determine the meaning of his/her fears, and re-examine his/her behavior. In other words, an empathic physician must sense, intuit and feel a patient's medical situation. To show empathy, the physician should feel genuinely sorry for the patient's medical predicament and do everything possible to comfort the patient. Some physicians believe that sympathy is sufficient to treat a terminally ill patient. I will argue that sympathy is insufficient to help a terminally ill patient deal with a negative diagnosis since it is not psychologically complex enough to show the patient that the physician really cares about the patient's medical situation. Empathy also shows the patient that the physician will care for him/her to the end.

Empathy is, therefore, essential for a humanistic encounter between physician and patient, since through empathy the physician can empathize with the patient's illness and his/her medical situation. Empathy can be characterized as a culmination of the above four conditions since if a physician treats his/her terminally ill patient dualistically in terms of the illness as it is experienced by a particular patient rather than as a diseased body, stressing the lived, subjective experience of illness by paying close attention to a terminally ill patient's clinical narrative, the physician is actively approaching the complex psychological state of empathy. Empathy is best understood as a device that will assist in the understanding of the other person--not merely the feelings of communion or fellow-feeling "along with" the other person, as would be the case with a sympathetic response to the other person.

The traditional paradigm of medicine views the terminally ill patient's illness as a diseased state of the body that could be cured using various kinds of treatment and/or surgery. For the physician, a disease state is an entity that can be separated from the person experiencing the illness. For the terminally ill patient, on the other hand, the illness is part of his/her body and affects his/her quality of life since it fundamentally affects his/her whole sense of personhood. The difference between the physician's conceptualization of illness as a disease and the patient's as a lived experience that affects every aspect of his/her existence highlights the reason why the patient and physician often discover how difficult it is to effectively communicate with one another. The patient-centered approach advocated in this book here prescribes ways that effective communication can be achieved.

Conclusion

In this chapter, I have examined how a physician could ensure that the terminally ill patient understands the information that (s)he discloses. The disclosure of a negative diagnosis is very difficult for a patient to accept without experiencing some initial shock or grief. This is a very natural response to a negative diagnosis; however, such a response complicates acceptance and understanding of the diagnosis. Thus, the physician and other medical staff must help the patient accept the diagnosis and determine what (s)he will do next given his/her medical predicament. Developing an effective physician and patient relationship is essential in enhancing understanding and the mutual trust and respect that results.

Chapter 6

Successful Decision-Making

In this chapter, I discuss the importance of shared decision-making between patient and physician when treating the terminally ill. Patients who suddenly become terminally ill may not be able to make rational decisions about their future medical treatments on their own. Thus, it is essential that the terminally ill patient make his/her decisions about treatments in conjunction with the physician. The physician's role is to guide the patient to make a rational decision about any future medical treatments. As was mentioned in the last chapter, a patient's decision-making capabilities may be biased because of the initial shock of hearing a negative diagnosis. Most individuals are in denial about death and find it difficult to accept that they may actually be seriously ill at any point. Everyone wants to believe that (s)he will always be healthy. This is an illusion since each of us will ultimately get seriously ill at some point in our lives and we will have to make some important choices about treatments.

This chapter will focus on what constitutes successful decision-making and how a physician could determine whether or not a terminally ill patient is making a rational decision about a medical treatment, given that many times, terminally ill patients become biased and make irrational decisions about which medical treatment is the most effective, because of the medical situation and their own vulnerabilities. When this occurs, the physician must ensure, through shared decision-making, that the terminally ill patient makes a rational decision. In this chapter, I will focus on several overarching aspects of successful decision-making which underlie the patient-centered approach to medicine that has been advocated throughout the book.

A rational decision may be defined as a decision that is consistent with a patient's values, goals, beliefs and life plans, one which is not influenced by biases and prejudices that are irrelevant to the decision being made. It is essential that physicians guide a patient's decision-making processes because of the possible effects of the medications.

If a terminally ill patient is on medication, this may debilitate his/her ability to think rationally. In such a case, the physician should either advise that the terminally ill patient stop taking the medication twelve, twenty four or even forty eight hours prior to making an important decision, and/or guide his/her decision-making processes by taking into account the expected psychological effects to ensure that the decision is rational. This condition of a patient-centered approach is much more complex than is apparent on the surface because sometimes a physician may have to guide the terminally ill patient's decision by unintentionally projecting some of his/her values, outcomes and conclusions onto the patient in a way that may seem paternalistic. According to the patient-centered model outlined throughout this book, any paternalistic decision-making is not permissible since it violates a patient's capacity for making rational and autonomous decisions about medical treatments. Physicians must therefore ensure that they are guiding the terminally ill patient but not prescribing what they consider the most beneficial treatments. To 'guide' means to 'think along with' the terminally ill patient, helping him/her to deliberate rationally and reflectively. This process is typically most effective when physicians keep asking the terminally ill patient relevant questions about the alternatives of treatment(s) discussed in order to ensure that (s)he has, in fact, understood them at each point of disclosure.

Patients who are terminally ill may experience continuous pain over a prolonged period of time and have often been prescribed mind altering and debilitating medication; it is for this reason that the physicians must devise special methodologies and procedures for handling such terminally ill patients. It is obvious, however, that physicians cannot always ensure that a rational decision is made by each terminally ill patient; however, if a patient has substantial self-knowledge, then the difficulty is manageable, and an informed consent could still be achieved. The difficulty is made almost impossible by terminally ill patients who lack self-knowledge.

There are four dimensions of rational decision-making: I. reflective deliberation; II. avoiding cognitive errors; III. reflective awareness; and IV. empathic understanding.

I. Reflective Deliberation

The successful achievement of reflective deliberation presupposes that the terminally ill patient has rationally evaluated his/her choice of treatments. To rationally deliberate about a treatment, one must not allow emotional and/or psychological influences an undue weight. This is a difficult stage of the deliberative process since when a patient is diagnosed with a terminal illness, (s)he feels vulnerable because of the continuous pain and other kinds of distress. There are ways that physicians can help such patients be more reflective by ensuring that errors in judgment do not occur. This is one of the tasks of the physician since without proper reflection the terminally ill patient may fail to give an informed consent.

II. Erroneous Cognitive Processes

In order to circumvent biases and errors of reasoning, it will be beneficial to consider some important and, at the same time, alarming findings conducted by two prominent cognitive psychologists, Kahneman and Tversky.[1] Errors in reasoning and judgment are not unusual when patients make decisions in favour of certain medical treatments due to the inherent vulnerabilities which are created by the medical setting. These errors of reasoning and judgment are responsible for some patients' inability to make a rational decision about a medical procedure. Erroneous beliefs play a key role in a patient's decision-making process since biased reasoning may arise while considering the information initially disclosed in the alternative treatments. Thus, the manner in which the patient interprets and internally represents the medical alternatives is crucially important. There are two possible errors of judgment under uncertainty: (i) belief bias effects; and (ii) framing effects.

(i) A "bias" may be defined as a systematic tendency to emphasize factors that are peripheral or irrelevant to the decision being made or to ignore factors that are strictly relevant. In order for a patient to capture the cognitive processes underlying decision-making, s(he) must become aware of the "biases" which may be consciously or unconsciously present when making decisions. For Tversky and Kahneman, "belief bias effects are defined as biases that patients have in "processing probability information". "Probability information" is roughly that which is needed for risk assessment.

In order to make a decision about whether to undergo a given medical intervention, terminally ill patients must reach judgments about the probability of certain outcomes. This perceived probability of outcomes is crucial for making an informed decision about a medical treatment. Research has been conducted to ascertain the processes that are involved in making decisions about probabilities. Kahneman and Tversky proposed two heuristics, namely, (a) representativeness; and (b) availability, which can be used by individuals in making decisions about probabilities.

(a) The "representative heuristic" influences and substantially biases a patient's decisions in ways that are unacceptable to autonomous decision-making. The representativeness heuristic results in a decision that is biased by previous decisions that are representative of the decision at hand. For instance, if the patient has undergone a previous medical treatment which was unsuccessful, painful, etc., his/her decision may be influenced by that previous instance and therefore (s)he will expect the previous treatment to be representative of the second one. Thus, the patient may erroneously decide against a medical treatment believing that it will be representative of the previous ones that failed, when in fact, this treatment may be successful in alleviating some, or all, of the misery that (s)he is experiencing. In this way, the patient may be led to errors and biases in his/her reasoning when (s)he, either consciously or unconsciously has internally represented the medical treatment in some biased manner.

(b) According to Tversky and Kahneman,[2] patients may also make decisions based on the probability that certain events can readily be brought to mind. Probabilities that occur frequently are usually recalled quicker and applied to the situation at hand, even if they are not strictly relevant to it. However, just because a certain event can be called to mind with greater ease that doesn't necessarily make it an effective basis for an accurate decision. In fact, if a patient decides about a given medical treatment too hastily without rationally considering all the risks and benefits, (s)he may be influenced by the availability heuristic since his/her decision was derived, not from careful evaluations and assessments of the information presented, but from a biased intuition that was immediately grasped without rational calculation. This often leads to irrational decision-making.

(ii) Framing Effects are characterized as the way in which information is presented by the physician and interpreted by the terminally ill patient who may formulate a personalized representation of the treatment and, because of the way such information is framed, may misinterpret the details of the treatments to fit his/her own framing projections and preferences. There are times when the terminally ill patient may be faced with high risk prospects in his/her treatment. If the physician communicates this high risk directly in his/her disclosure of the treatment, then the terminally ill patient may 'frame' the intervention solely in terms of the risks involved rather than the benefits or, alternatively, only in terms of the successes rather than risks. For instance, if a terminally ill patient perceives the options of surgery in terms of the probabilities of survival, this kind of "framing" may hinder the patient from simultaneously being able to perceive or understand the risk of death.

There are two ways in which terminally ill patients may unconsciously deal with risky information. First, the terminally ill patient may be in a state of denial about the severity of his/her illness and may engage in wishful thinking which is self-deceptive and may interfere with autonomous decision-making. For instance, a survival "frame" may prevent a patient from grasping that there may be a risk of death during the surgery. It is essential that the terminally ill patient, if (s)he is to give a properly informed consent to undergo a particular medical treatment, does not bias a treatment alternative. Every individual, prior to getting terminally ill, has the ultimate hope that (s)he will live for quite a long time. Yet when serious illness threatens an individual's life span and well being, his/her sense of integrity and personhood is severely undermined, and (s)he usually finds it difficult to make a rational choice if s(he) is not reflective, disciplined, and resolute about the medical situation and the treatments available.

Second, a terminally ill patient may process the risk or inevitability of death due to illness by "framing" the treatments in terms of the risks of uncertainty. When dealing with risky treatment such as a bone-Marrow transplant or chemotherapy for cancer patients, the choices available to the patient may have both negative and uncertain results. The patient may have to make a decision between either prolonging his/her life by undergoing surgery, and perhaps prolonging pain and misery or not engaging in any treatment and accepting death in the near future. Is it rational for cancer patients to refuse treatment? This is a difficult question to answer objectively since it depends on an individual's preferences and rationally calculated judgments. Naturally, the final decision depends on the patient's beliefs and values. If a patient strongly believes in the sanctity of life, (s)he may opt for surgery and prolonging life, despite some of the later difficulties. However, if the patient believes in dying with dignity, (s)he may opt for minimizing the time (s)he must suffer with pain and uncertainty. As long as the patient's decision is consistent with his/her life-long values, beliefs, and goals, and not made on irrational impulse or fear, the patient has a right to decide for himself/herself.

III. Reflective Awareness

Reflective Awareness is a process through which the mind becomes aware of its own operations. A more practical characterization is that reflective awareness is a process of examining our thinking processes, trying, for example, to determine how we derived our initial assessments. In order to achieve this, we must become introspective about our own thinking processes to retrace our initial deliberations. The terms 'introspective', 'reflective' and 'deliberative' have distinctive meanings and should not be conflated or considered to mean more or less the same. Deliberative processes consist of our first-order, ordinary pre-reflective thinking, which has already been examined above. In introspection, an individual must become aware of his/her own thinking processes that made up those deliberative first-order processes. Introspection is a process that makes it possible to be aware of ordinary, first-order deliberation and second order, reflective awareness. The evaluative stage of the awareness occurs at the reflective, second-order stage when the individual makes a judgment about the thinking processes. In other words, there is a level distinction between ordinary, first order awareness and reflection, which is assessment and evaluation of what one has thought or experienced.

Thus, reflective awareness is a second-order deliberative process, which requires that the patient evaluate his/her initial decisions of medical treatments, and the alternatives s(he) initially chose. The process of reflective awareness is somewhat difficult to understand as it is usually described using phenomenological language. Reflective awareness is generally defined as a type of conscious, second-order reflection, and some individuals may have difficulty adequately incorporating it into their decision-making methods. Some individuals may find it difficult to grasp the meaning of what constitutes second-order reflection, which is a form of introspection or 'turning back' on our initial interpretations. This state of mind or attitude is quite distinct from our ordinary, everyday pre-reflective deliberative processes, which is the foundation for reflective awareness.

Reflective awareness substantially contributes to the success of a patient's making a rational decision about a medical treatment; it ensures that the patient will critically evaluate all the medical information disclosed by the physician and make certain than this decision is consistent with his/her values, beliefs and life goals. This process will also ensure that the decision is both rational and autonomous. This evaluative analysis takes a considerable amount of time to achieve and depends on the terminally ill patient. Different individuals have different capacities for second-order reflection, and not every person is equally reflective. In addition, since illness and medication may weaken a terminally ill patient's reflective capacities, this may result in extending the process even longer. For individuals that are psychologically debilitated by illness or medication, the reflective process must be attempted two or more times in order to determine whether their initial reflective evaluations were accurate.

Thus, reflective awareness signifies more than the freedom to choose between alternative modes of medical treatment. It requires that a terminally ill patient makes a reflective choice that represents his/her deeply held beliefs and preferences, not those of a brief or fleeting duration. The patient must seek out those beliefs that are permanent and stable parts of his/her life experiences. Terminally ill patients are more than a bundle of individual behaviours; they are capable of reflective awareness which ensures that their decisions will carefully calculated and thus morally autonomous.

When reflective awareness is effective, the physician will not be subject to nearly as much uncertainty in obtaining a rational decision in favor of a medical procedure. It will be possible to be much more confident in determining whether the terminally ill patient has adequately understood the information which was disclosed, and whether his/her decision was influenced by other irrelevant considerations. The physician can do this by being attentive to the kinds of questions that the terminally ill patient asks and the kind of clarifications that (s)he believes are critical to his/her making a proper decision. Most terminally ill patients will make decisions that are consistent with the type of individuals that they are, and if the physician has an intuition of this fact, s(he) will have added confidence in assessing whether his/her terminally ill patient has in fact made a rational and autonomous decision.

But what if the physician, while disclosing the information about a medical treatment to his/her terminally ill patient, recognizes that (s)he lacks adequate rational, reflective deliberation and simply decides about a particular treatment in an unreflective manner? Does the physician have a duty to probe further in order to enable his/her terminally ill patient to comprehend all the information presented in a reflective manner? On the patient-centered model, reflective deliberation is a central moral requirement of rational decision-making and of an informed consent, and the physician does therefore have a moral duty to ensure that a patient's decisions are autonomous and calculative in nature, provided that the patient has adequate self-knowledge and is only temporarily debilitated. The physician could help the patient further reflect by guiding and encouraging the terminally ill patient's thinking processes to reflect as deeply as possible on the risks and benefits of the alternative treatments in order to ensure that the patient's decision is ultimately rational and autonomous. Some medical practitioners may be critical of this view and respond by saying that this is placing an unwarranted burden on the physician, that it is not the physician's responsibility to ensure that a rational decision is made. Instead, it is the patient's prerogative to make certain that his/her decisions are autonomous. But while most patients can make autonomous decisions, some patients need more guidance from medical practitioners in order to make rational and reflective decisions about future medical treatments.

IV. Empathic Understanding

One of the most important features of patient-centered health care is for the physician to ensure that the patient gives a proper consent for treatment. From a personal perspective, the terminally ill patient may be depressed about his/her illness and in constant pain. Empathy can help a physician detect many forms of psychological distress, and to prescribe antidepressants to help some terminally ill patients cope so that they could give a proper consent in the future. If such psychological distress goes untreated, it could cause a terminally ill patient to become prematurely despondent about his/her medical situation. Thus, it is important for the physician to sufficiently get to know the terminally ill patient in order to determine whether or not his/her depression should be treated before (s)he makes a decision in favor of a treatment.[3] This is the interpersonal component of obtaining an informed consent for a treatment. Through an empathetic understanding of the terminally ill patient's situation and by developing a relationship of mutual trust and respect with him/her, the physician could determine whether or not (s)he should help the patient choose the best treatment. Below, I outline five guidelines that physicians should use to ensure that a terminally ill patient gives an informed consent for a treatment. As will be shown, empathy is the foundation of each of these guidelines.

First, a physician must gain a sufficient amount of knowledge of the terminally ill patient, not only in terms of his/her medical history but as a unique person. This process involves becoming aware of the patient's beliefs, values, desires, long and short-term goals, principles, moral and/or religious inclinations. In addition, it is essential that the physician gain a sufficient amount of information about the patient's temperament, character traits, and attitudes. For instance, the physician should be aware of whether or not the patient is predominantly happy, unhappy, sad, content, and in a happy or unhappy marriage and so on.[4] Such psychological attitudes and states of affairs can have a negative impact on a patient's outlook, and this is especially the case when the patient becomes terminally ill since such an individual will usually develop a cynical attitude towards himself/herself and life in general and will be increasingly prone to experiencing even more negative emotions because (s)he is in constant pain. Thus, through an empathetic understanding of the patient's attitudes before illness, the physician can monitor and assess the terminally ill patient's attitudes. The more the physician strives to gain an understanding of the patient, the more empathetic will the physician become with the patient's medical situation.

Second, the decision in favor of a treatment must be made by the patient in collaboration with the physician. The terminally ill patient should always clearly communicate his/her medical needs to the physician. It is essential that the physician become reflexively aware of the patient's medical concerns and any familial idiosyncrasies, such as whether there is a manipulative spouse, financial difficulties, and so on. Relatives or family should not become the sole decision makers on behalf of patients since there is ample evidence in the literature that they do not always genuinely know the terminally ill patient or what is in his/her best interest.[5] Studies indicate that families only correctly predict a patient's treatment preferences in sixty to seventy percent of cases.[6] It is essential that the physician knows as much as possible about the terminally ill patient's life and psychological health. Sometimes relatives may bias a terminally ill patient's decision by manipulating him/her into believing that (s)he is a financial and psychological burden to other family members because of his/her illness. Other times, relatives may project their negative feelings of uncertainty and vulnerability onto the patient, who is already feeling vulnerable because of prolonged pain and discomfort. Still other times, a patient may not want to endure a particular treatment prematurely because of negative comments uttered by relatives.[7] Physicians must avoid such difficulties by developing a relationship of mutual trust and respect with the patient. In cases of terminal illness, medical decision-making is a long and continuous process. Informed consent will take the form of shared decision-making which is one of the manifestations of a genuinely informed consent.[8]

Third, the physician should help the patient create an advanced personal policy statement outlining his/her long-term intentions about matters of health.[9] An advanced personal policy statement is usually regarded as advanced decision-making since the patient decides what (s)he will do if (s)he becomes terminally ill. The process of creating an advanced statement also allows the physician to empathetically understand the patient's beliefs, values, goals and plans, which will allow the physician to become aware of the patient's life plans should (s)he become terminally ill. Some patients want the kind of terminal care that emphasizes palliative care. Other patients will want direct, open assistance in the termination of their lives. Still other patients may want other options in between. It is essential that the patient make a decision based on his/her long-term beliefs, values, principles, and moral and/religious priorities. The physician can help the patient collaboratively make such important decisions by empathically talking about the alternatives, and determining with the patient which option would be the best for him/her, given his/her situation. By creating an advanced personal policy statement, a patient will ensure that when the time comes to make a decision about whether or not to endure a particular treatment, and (s)he is unable to rationally do so, that his/her autonomy will not be violated by family members, relatives, or other third parties. Such a policy statement also protects against slippery slope difficulties.[10] This also gives the physician peace of mind should the patient eventually need to determine whether or not to end his/her life. I will focus on creating advanced policy statements in more detail in Chapter 8.

Fourth, the patient's request for treatment must be continuous, conscious, reflective and freely made. There is so much room for abuse in this area that it is essential that a physician empathically communicate directly with the terminally ill patient to ensure that (s)he is making a decision that is rational, informed, and his/her own, one which is unbiased by relatives and family, or his/her own negative psychological states. If the patient feels pressured, (s)he should stand back for a while before making a decision. If the patient is depressed, (s)he should be prescribed antidepressants, and (s)he should wait a while before making a decision. In this way, the physician could strive to be empathically responsive to the patient's needs, in the administration of humane health care. However, if the patient makes continuous and consistent requests in favor of a particular treatment, and (s)he is rational, not forced, biased or depressed, then his/her request is genuine.

Fifth, the physician must empathically determine whether or not the patient's pain and suffering cannot be relieved by other means. Sometimes there are other medical treatments for a patient. For example, a terminally ill patient's illness may not be progressing quickly; thus, prescribing stronger pain medication may be the answer. Other times, it may be necessary to prescribe morphine so that the patient will not be in as much discomfort. A physician must be empathetic with the patient's terminal illness, pain, and suffering by imagining what it would be like to be in the patient's predicament. The physician must ask himself, "How would I feel if I was in so much pain?" Sometimes, a patient may feel that (s)he should end his/her life because of extreme pain and suffering. Giving a terminally ill patient more pain medication in such a situation could be considered an empathetic course of action since the physician may feel that the patient could be more comfortable. Some physicians resist prescribing medication to terminally ill patients because they do not want the patient to get addicted to narcotics.[11] This is an unnecessary precaution and it does not usually exhibit empathy towards a patient who is in severe pain.

Conclusion

Rational and shared decision-making is especially important for the patient who must make a decision about his/her health. Many times, patients may make decisions which are counterintuitive and biased. Thus, the physician should always determine if the patient should be helped to make important decisions. This does not mean that the physician must make a decision on the terminally ill patient's behalf. The physician's role is merely to 'guide' the patient's thinking processes so that (s)he could make a rational decision that is free from biases. Thus, the physician merely plays the role of mentor and collaborator of decision-making. Some physicians still resist shared decision-making because of the psychological complexity that is involved in such situations. However, shared decision-making can sometimes save a terminally ill patient's life and ensure that (s)he is making a rational decision about future interventions.

Thus, physicians may need to spend a substantial amount of time guiding some of their patients' thinking processes. Some terminally ill patients may lack the second-order reflective awareness that is necessary to make assessments about previously made decisions. The physician should not expect the terminally ill patient to proceed on his or her own since, given their medical condition, that patient may lack proper second order reflection in order to make a rational decision. This requires that the physician and terminally ill patient engage in effective communication in order to reach a rational decision about a medical intervention together. Effective communication, in turn, requires that an effective physician-patient relationship is developed and nurtured.

Chapter 7

Effective Communication

The purpose of this chapter is to discuss the importance of effective communication with a terminally ill patient. A patient-centered approach cannot be achieved unless a physician empathically understands a patient's medical predicament and can communicate openly and honestly. These two cognitive processes take a substantial amount of time to develop. In the process, the physician should strive to get to know the patient and his/her personal and medical preferences as quickly as possible. One way to foster an effective physician-patient relationship is by developing mutual trust and respect. It is never appropriate for a physician to merely manipulate a terminally ill patient into agreeing to undergo a particular treatment since this stifles open, honest communication.

Effective communication is also one of the building blocks for developing an effective physician-patient relationship. The relationship itself becomes complex due to the intrinsic vulnerabilities of medicine and the patient's terminal illness. In this chapter, I will focus on the essential features of effective communication between the physician and patient which ensure that a patient gives an informed decision in favor of or against a treatment. The thesis of this chapter is that effective communication is impossible to achieve without adhering to certain principles of honesty and, without these, the terminally ill patient cannot give a proper consent. Honesty is the bedrock of all significant relationships, and this is no less the case between the physician and a terminally ill patient.

There are three conditions of effective communication: (1) Honesty; (2) Promise-keeping/confidentiality; and (3) Caring and empathy. To this end, the chapter will be divided into three main parts. In Part I, I discuss honesty and its importance for effective communication. Honesty is the overarching virtue in this triad since without it, the other two conditions lose their ultimate significance. If a physician and terminally ill patient are honest with one another, there is a high probability that they will communicate effectively and develop a rapport of trust and respect with one another. In Part II, I discuss the importance of promise-keeping and confidentiality in physician-patient encounters. When a patient becomes ill, it is essential for the physician to keep his/her promises with the patient. In Part III, I discuss the importance of empathy in developing effective communication between physician and the patient. An empathic physician imagines what it would be like to endure the patient's continuous pain, distress and suffering. Being empathetic in this way will give the physician a proper appreciation of the terminally ill patient's discomfort and anxiety level. Empathic appreciation also enhances the ability of the physician to effectively communicate with a terminally ill patient.

I. Honesty

Honesty is a complex notion which has a multitude of possible psychological, moral, and religious connotations all of which may change the meaning of the term for each particular patient according to the context in which the word is used. Generally, a physician or patient is honest if s(he) is fair and sincere in both his/her personal character and behaviour, and is not deceitful or untrustworthy. In this section, I examine two kinds of honesty: (1) physician honesty; and (2) patient honesty.[1]

(1) Physician honesty consists of an adequate description of the diagnosis and alternative treatments available to the terminally ill patient, proper disclosure of the information in terms that can be understood by him/her, the prudence not to bias a terminally ill patient's response in favour of certain treatment(s), and the avoidance of intentional deception through exaggerations or lies such as: "If you don't undergo treatment X, you will surely die". These characteristics of honesty should be carefully considered by physicians to ensure that an honest exchange with the patient will result.

Avoiding intentionally deceiving patients is perhaps the most important concern to address since it is not uncommon for physicians to engage in disingenuousness about a particular medical alternative without saying anything that is explicitly or strictly speaking false.[2] The situation of deliberate deceit is not generally distinct from lying since if the physician intends to deceive, s(he) intended to lie, and therefore the physician's action would be considered morally wrong since deception of this kind undermines a patient's autonomy and right to make a decision based on a disclosure of all the known treatments and their risks and benefits. The American Medical Association's "Principles of Ethics" of 1980 insists that the physician "deal honestly with patients and colleagues and strive to expose those physicians deficient in character or competence, or who engage in fraud and deception."[3]

Two types of dishonesty are prevalent in the physician-patient relationship: (i) Deception; and (ii) Lying.[4]

(i) A is deceived by B if B persuades A of something that is false or B purposefully misleads A into thinking something is the case when in fact it is not. Most of the deception that is morally wrong in the medical setting is voluntary in nature. The act of deception has three elements: (a) evasion; (b) digression; and (c) distortion.

(a) Evasion occurs when Person B diverts Person A's attention to another issue which is irrelevant to the main issue, so that A will be led to believe differently as a result. Evasion also occurs when, for example, there is a failure to directly answer a terminally ill patient's queries by leading him/her to believe that the question was not important or by focusing on a similar question that fails to directly address some of the terminally ill patient's main concerns.

(b) Digression occurs when Person B intentionally focuses on another aspect of the situation instead of focusing on what Person A is strictly concerned with. This kind of response is disrespectful since it inadvertently gives the message that the patient's opinion is not worth the physician's consideration. In any effective physician-patient exchange, the patient's opinion is crucially important, and should never be dismissed.

(c) Distortion occurs when Person B reinterprets the facts initially understood by Person A and expresses them in a way that is ambiguous or vague in relation to Person A's initial interpretation. Such a response fails to acknowledge the terminally ill patient's concerns by undermining his/her interpretations of his/her bodily states. A physician must never, under any circumstances, pretend that his/her interpretation of the medical situation is more accurate than the patient's.

These three forms of deception are morally wrong since they undermine the possibility of achieving a patient-centered approach to medicine. Within this model, it can never be permissible to intentionally or unintentionally use deceptive techniques when communicating the medical alternatives to a terminally ill patient. If a physician is aware of a gap in the patient's medical knowledge, this fact should be honestly communicated to him/her. Any form of deception erodes the possibility of developing an effective physician-patient relationship. However, some forms of deception may be unintentional in that the physician may not intend to deceive a terminally ill patient.

(ii) Lying is a direct utterance of a false statement. It occurs when messages are communicated to another individual with the intention of misleading him/her and to make the person believe as true what the other individual believes is false. In short, to lie is to persuade someone to hold a false belief as if it were true. False statements are usually made to undermine a patient's interpretation of the medical facts. A physician who lies to a terminally ill patient is operating under the old traditional, paternalistic view of the physician-patient relationship where (s)he believes that lying is justified in order to get the patient to agree with a particular treatment. Such a paternalistic attitude obviously undermines the patient's autonomy, and the consent that the patient gives under such conditions can never be informed. To build an effective relationship that is based on mutual trust and respect, the physician must honour the patient's self-determination.

In addition, when a physician intentionally lies to a patient, s(he) is undermining that patient's basic human right to decide which treatments to try, given his/her medical situation. Every patient has a right to receive a disclosure of all the alternative treatments, including all the risks and benefits. A physician who intentionally withholds such medical information from a terminally ill patient does not respect his/her autonomy, and stifles any possibility of experiencing open, honest, communication that can lead to mutual trust and respect. Only a closely knit physician-patient relationship could survive all the vulnerabilities created by the medical situation in which illness, pain, and suffering dominate the relation.

2. The terminally ill patient also has a duty to be honest with the physician since the relationship is based on a reciprocality of mutual trust and respect. Most patients are not intentionally dishonest with their physicians since such dishonesty is not in their best interest. However, due to the vulnerabilities caused by the terminality of a disease, and the pain and suffering that accrues as a result, the patient may sometimes exaggerate either the symptoms or the pain and suffering that (s)he is enduring. This is the case when an illness makes a terminally ill patient feel overly anxious. Once a certain set of facts are communicated to the physician, (s)he must respond on the basis of the patient's assessment of these facts. If this assessment is not firmly grounded in reality, the physician will not have an accurate description of the patient's experience of illness. To get around this possibility, the physician must ensure, through further questioning and discussion with the terminally ill patient, that the patient is not over or underestimating his/her medical condition. This procedure is also beneficial to the patient since s(he) is given a reality check about his/her experience of illness. In this way, the patient is usually able to step back from the symptoms and decide for him/herself whether or not his/her initial assessment was accurate.

Effective communication is impossible to achieve without an honest exchange between physician and patient. Neither can mutual trust and respect be fostered without open, honest communication. The purpose of communication is substantially undermined when one person intentionally engages in deception. To communicate means, in principle, to convey true but not false or misleading information in order to evoke understanding, and to transmit feelings and emotions to an individual. There is no point in conveying false information to another person since it is assumed by most individuals that the information disclosed will be true unless the patient proves to be untrustworthy.

II. Promise-Keeping/Confidentiality

If the terminally ill patient cannot assume that the physician will keep information about his/her health confidential, the patient may not feel comfortable about disclosing important information to the physician, and open, honest communication will be stifled, if not destroyed. Thus, promise-keeping is an important aspect for building a physician-patient relationship that is based on mutual trust and respect. There are two kinds of promise-keeping: (i) physician confidentiality; and (ii) patient confidentiality.[5]

(i) When a terminally ill patient discloses personal information about himself/herself, s(he) expects that the physician will not break his/her implicit promise to keep the information confidential. The physician has a duty not to disclose personal information about his/her patient to relatives, friends, or colleagues, without the patient's express permission.[6] When a physician breaches the patient's trust in this way, the relationship may be either damaged or completely ruined, depending on the kind of information that was disclosed. For some terminally ill patients, even a one time breach of trust will put the relationship in jeopardy since that trust that is an implicit part of the relationship will be undermined.

The most important breach of physician confidentiality occurs when relatives insist that they be given important information about the patient because they feel that they have a right to know. Some physicians would argue that this should not be considered a breach of confidentiality since information is disclosed to close relatives and not to strangers. However, it can be rightfully argued that any personal information disclosed about a patient to any third party (close relatives or complete strangers) without the express permission of the patient must be considered a breach of trust. The physician's primary responsibility is to the patient and not to his/her relatives. The mere communication between the physician and a relative without a patient's physical presence is dishonest, and breaks the trust between the two individuals. Consider the following case:

> Nancy White, a 57 year old mother of two was admitted to the hospital to rule out breast cancer. Despite Nancy's apparent pain, she appeared to be a well-balanced and rational individual. This was especially apparent when the physician diagnosed her health condition, and the possibility of cancer. Nancy was reflective about the whole testing procedure and wanted to know whether she had cancer so that, if she did, she could take the necessary steps to stop the spread of the disease. While the tests were being processed, Nancy's husband and daughters approached the physician and asked him to disclose the results of the tests to them before telling Nancy. The relatives told the physician that Nancy was unable to handle bad news due to her fear of cancer. They

further said that Nancy had been mentally distressed since she began feeling sick and they would appreciate it if the physician would disclose the test results to them first. The tests came back positive. What should the physician do?

It is obvious that Nancy has manipulative relatives. Nancy showed no sign of mental distress when the physician spoke to her. In fact, she exhibited no fears whatsoever, making it seem that these fears were projections derived from Nancy's family. In spite of this fact, the physician has no implicit or explicit duty to disclose such information to relatives without the patient's express permission. The physician must, therefore, disclose the test results to Nancy first, and tell her about her relatives concern for knowing whether or not she had cancer. If Nancy should then ask the physician to tell her relatives, then the physician would be required to do so. Otherwise, it is Nancy's prerogative whether or not she tells her relatives; however, it is not the physician's duty to make such decisions.

Another way of ensuring that a patient is confident in the physician's honesty is for all third parties to speak to the physician about the patient in his/her presence. This helps to build patient trust and ensures that the patient decides how much personal information to disclose to relatives. The physician should never decide how much information to disclose on his/her own. In the patient's absence, the physician should not disclose any personal information to relatives. Any such breach of confidentiality is not permissible if effective communication is to result between the physician and patient.

There is an implicit moral relationship between physician and patient, and the confidentiality issue highlights this relationship sharply. The physician must act on the principle of fidelity by being loyal to the patient above all else. This aspect of a physician-patient relationship may seem controversial since one may ask: "Why does the physician have a duty to be morally bound to the patient?" The answer is quite obvious: Fidelity to a patient's concerns is necessary since an honest and forthright relationship cannot be built without securing a patient's confidential information. In addition, effective communication is enhanced if a physician is loyal to the patient.

(ii) The physician must also trust that the terminally ill patient will keep certain medical information confidential. These may be facts about the uncertainties of certain treatments or some yet experimental methods of treatment. In an effective physician-patient relationship, the physician may disclose information about gaps in his/her medical knowledge, fears that the outcome of certain treatments are more risky than others, and confidence about administering certain treatments over others. The physician expects that the patient will keep such information confidential. Thus, the physician and patient are morally bound to one another in a manner that should keep all third parties extrinsic to their relationship. This is the only way to ensure that an effective physician-patient relationship will be secure, amidst the typical vulnerabilities of a terminal illness, and the problem of close relatives possibly infringing on the patient's personal boundaries.

III. Caring and Empathy

Empathy involves reflecting on the terminally ill patient's feelings, emotions and medical situation, and presupposes an intensity and distinct type of active/interactive response on the part of the physician. One important feature of empathy is being in "communion" or "synchrony" with another individual. The empathizer (i.e., the physician) can initially better understand what the patient is experiencing by his/her verbal reports and body language. The physician can apprehend the patient's medical situation if: s(he) has already experienced the medical condition first-hand, has seen someone close to him/her (such as a family member or friend) experience a similar medical situation second-hand, and can form a mental representation or analogue of the situation. One or more of the three conditions are necessary if the physician is to effectively empathize with the patient, since empathy is imaginatively reflecting on "what it would be like" to be in the patient's medical situation.

If a physician genuinely cares about the patient, s(he) will be empathetic with his/her pain, suffering, and vulnerabilities. By being empathetic, the physician will be able to put him/herself in the patient's shoes, and ask "What would it be like if I had the terminal illness my patient is enduring?" In this way, the physician will be able to better understand the patient's predicament and more effectively communicate with the patient. Without an empathetic attitude towards the patient, the physician-patient relationship remains strictly professional, stifling the interpersonal interaction that is necessary for the patient to properly understand the treatment alternatives available. The patient must feel comfortable with his/her physician in order to ask any questions (s)he may have about the treatments without the physician being judgmental.

A continuing theme of the book has been that the physician should strive to understand the patient interpersonally by becoming cognizant of the patient's values, goals, beliefs, long and short term goals, and personal character traits. Such an appreciation of the patient's personal self is only possible by developing an empathetic, caring and responsible relationship with him/her, one that will allow the patient's personal idiosyncrasies to emerge. The patient must feel that the physician is treating him/her as a unique person and not merely a diseased body. To treat the whole patient, the physician must recognize the patient's personal idiosyncrasies and accept them uncritically, and to be acutely aware of the way illness and disease causes inherent vulnerabilities in all human beings. These vulnerabilities could be lessened by the physician through an empathetic interaction with the patient. The physician must feel that s(he) can be of assistance to his/her terminally ill patient in a way that transcends medical boundaries and reaches inside the patient's own idiosyncrasies.

An empathetic attitude towards a patient may also facilitate recovery or remission from an illness. An empathetic physician is usually able to positively encourage a terminally ill patient by empowering him/her to take the necessary small steps on the path to recovery from surgery or other painful treatments. The terminally ill patient must feel that the physician genuinely wants him/her to progressively get healthier. Such a positive and encouraging attitude is crucial for a terminally ill patient to recover quickly.

Conclusion

The physician-patient relationship is unique since the two individuals usually enter into it voluntarily. At the beginning of the relationship, the physician is usually regarded as a professional who will alleviate pain and suffering or give medical advice to a patient. Thus, there appears to be an inequality of power between the two parties at the beginning of the relationship in that the patient is dependent on the physician for medical advice. If the relationship is to become more mature, however, the structure of the relationship must fundamentally change from a relationship of unequals to one of equals. This will ensure that the physician and patient communicate openly and honestly with one another. The physician must recognize that his/her terminally ill patient is a person whose bodily functions are permanently incapacitated by illness and is in need of medical advice. However, the terminally ill patient's sense of autonomy should not be undermined, although the patient's ability to make autonomous decisions may be weakened because of the illness. The physician must always assume that the patient is capable of making autonomous decisions, unless (s)he proves otherwise. Without effective communication, the patient would be unable to understand his/her treatment alternatives in order to rationally and effectively decide in favour of or against them. Thus, effective communication is one of the cornerstones of the patient-centered approach.

Chapter 8

Developing Effective Physician-Patient Relationships

To develop and nurture an effective physician-patient relationship, the physician must have an awareness of the terminally ill patient's beliefs, values, and life goals. The physician must also become aware of the patient as a person and not merely a diseased body that needs medical attention. Every terminally ill patient will have different needs for information-disclosure, depending on personal idiosyncrasies, and unless the physician is aware of these differences in advance, (s)he will not be able to effectively disclose the relevant information about possible treatments to the patient. Likewise, the terminally ill patient must also be cognizant of some of the physician's personal attitudes. For instance, if a physician has a habit of being hasty and impatient, s(he) will most probably not take the time to convey the relevant information about all aspects of the treatments. Open and honest communication between physician and the terminally ill patient is difficult to develop and maintain if the physician does not disclose all the details of the treatments to the patient. To develop an effective physician-patient relationship, the patient must trust that the physician has disclosed all the information about the treatments available, and the physician must trust that the patient has understood and rationally assessed all the relevant medical information. This reciprocal relationship of trust is one of the building blocks for an effective physician-patient relationship.

There are two centrally important features of an effective physician-patient relationship: effective disclosure, and shared decision-making. In Part I, I focus on effective disclosure and I will illustrate the difficulties with using manipulative techniques to communicate the medical treatments to the terminally ill patient. In Part II, I argue that shared decision-making is impossible to achieve without honest, open, and non-manipulative communication between patient and physician. Further, a physician who uses manipulative techniques erodes the possibility of developing an effective physician-patient relationship.

I. Effective Disclosure

For effective disclosure to occur, the exchange between physician and terminally ill patient must be free from the use of manipulative influences. Such irrational influences on the part of the physician may lead to falsely orchestrated decisions that are not substantially informed. In order to avoid irrational influences, the alternatives of treatment must be presented to the patient in an objective manner (i.e., free from psychological manipulations) and by taking the patient's beliefs, values and life goals into account. There are four kinds of manipulation:

(1) coercion;
(2) persuasion;
(3) prioritizing of information; and
(4) tone of voice.

(1) Coercion is defined as an intentional influence that exaggerates a credible threat of unwanted and avoidable harm that is so great that the terminally ill patient cannot resist acting to avoid it. In such a case, the terminally ill patient would be consenting to treatment that is not necessarily in his/her best interest. This occurs most notably when the physician is dogmatically convinced that the patient should undergo a given treatment without taking the patient's beliefs, values, and life goals into account. If the patient unreflectively accepts a particular treatment, s(he) is not making an autonomous decision in favour of that treatment.

Very few physicians use coercive techniques due to peer pressure and the irrational responses that are produced in the terminally ill patient. Physicians may unintentionally use coercion only as a last resort if they believe that the terminally ill patient is refusing treatment that (s)he should at least try. For instance, if it is recommended that a terminally ill patient undergo exploratory surgery and yet (s)he irrationally decides against it, the physician may try to coerce the patient by saying: "If you don't have exploratory surgery, you may not live for long". This tactic may also used to convince the patient to agree to undergo exploratory surgery as the quickest way of determining the extent and spread of the disease. In other words, by undergoing exploratory surgery a terminally ill patient often gains a peace of mind. However, even if a terminally ill patient makes an irrational decision against such surgery, the physician should resist using coercive techniques to convince him/her to undergo surgery. Instead, the physician should attempt to 'guide' the terminally ill patient's thinking so that s(he) will make a much more rational decision the second time the information about the treatments is disclosed. Some terminally ill patients make decisions in favour of treatments that are initially considered to be irrational, yet upon the second or third consideration of the treatments, such patients may become convinced that their previous decision was irrational.

(2) Persuasion may be characterized as the successful attempt to convince a terminally ill patient, through appeals to reason or emotion, in favour of a treatment that the physician believes (s)he should undergo in order to improve his/her overall medical situation. When a terminally ill patient's beliefs are manipulated by the physician, (s)he is persuaded to undergo a medical treatment that may not be in accordance with the moral autonomy and integrity of that patient. This is the most problematic of the two types of manipulation since it is sometimes difficult for the terminally ill patient to correctly ascertain whether or not (s)he is being persuasively influenced by the physician. Sometimes the physician may persuade the terminally ill patient so subtlely that the patient is completely unaware of being persuaded, and therefore, (s)he remains unreflectively aware of whether his/her decision was informed and autonomous or uninformed and non-autonomous.

(3) The priority with which the physician presents the treatments may also be significant to the patient. Terminally ill patients are sometimes influenced by the ordering of the medical treatments since they believe that the information that the physician presents first must involve the most beneficial (i.e., painless and relatively risk-free) treatments. The physician can, therefore, inadvertently manipulate the terminally ill patient by presenting what (s)he believes to be the most viable treatment first, such that by the time the physician discloses the third or fourth treatment, the patient may have reached his/her cognitive saturation point and is unable to remember what was previously disclosed. Therefore, the terminally ill patient would opt for the treatment (s)he remembers most clearly. One solution to such a quandary would be for the terminally ill patient to simply ask whether there is any importance attached to the ordering of the treatments. Another possible way to circumvent such difficulties would be for the terminally ill patient to ask that the treatments be written so that (s)he could read all of them over. This ensures that the terminally ill patient could study all the recommendations, not just the one the physician believes to be the primary treatment.

(4) Tone of voice can also be a powerful manipulative technique and must be avoided by the physician so that it does not give the terminally ill patient any way of misinterpreting the information. For instance, if a physician raises his/her voice while disclosing the treatment, this may give the terminally ill patient a feeling of uneasiness towards the treatment. In other cases, loud voices could imply that the physician is being authoritative about which treatment is best for the patient; this may again result in a patient's unreflective acceptance of a treatment. Thus, terminally ill patients may interpret loud or soft voices in a variety of non-rational ways, depending on their state of vulnerability.

Within the patient-centered model, it is never acceptable for physicians to use any type of manipulative techniques to convince terminally ill patients to decide in favour of a treatment, since such a pretense undermines a patient's autonomy, and ultimately erodes the physician-patient relationship. Such manipulative techniques also reinforce the much outmoded paternalistic model of medicine in which the physician prescribes a treatment without the patient's consent since the physician wrongly assumes that s(he) knows what is in the patient's best interest. Consent under the traditional model focused on harm-avoidance above all else, even if it meant undermining a patient's autonomy. On the patient-centered model, any consent that is given by a terminally ill patient must be autonomous. Thus, it is never appropriate for the physician to undermine the terminally ill patient's basic right of determining which treatment to endure for him/herself.

The physician could avoid these manipulative techniques by being especially prudent about how (s)he communicates the treatments to the terminally ill patient. In some cases, physicians might have to guide the terminally ill patient's thinking processes so that (s)he makes a rational, reflective and autonomous decision in favour or against a treatment. This is especially the case if the terminally ill patient is in considerable pain or on medication that may affect his/her thinking processes. However, 'guiding' should not mean 'deciding' on the patient's behalf, and then using manipulative techniques to convince him/her that s(he) must accept a particular treatment because it is in "the patient's best interest". It is, instead, the physician's duty to ensure that the terminally ill patient makes a rational, reflective, and well understood decision in favour of a treatment.

Many physicians use manipulative techniques without being consciously aware of them since they are an inherent part of the fabric of the traditional model of medicine. Some of the common justifications for using manipulative techniques are:

(i)   time constraints;
(ii)   deficiency in a patient's psychological competency; [1]
(iii) lack of physician patience;
(iv)   the patient's failure to understand technical medical terminology; and
(v)   character clashes. [2]

(i) It is always possible for physicians to make a case for being overworked and overstressed due to the everyday pressures and long hours of work that are a fundamental part of a physician's professional life. Physicians may feel overburdened by too many patients, an insufficient number of medical personnel, and long hours at the hospital and office. However, despite this, it is never justified for a physician to undermine a patient's autonomy and basic right to make a decision for him/herself due to time constraints, except in justified emergency situations.

(ii) Every terminally ill patient has a different level of intellectual and emotional perspicuity. The physician should become aware of the terminally ill patient's educational level before disclosing information about the treatments. Most patients are psychologically competent to make their own decisions about a medical treatment. The few terminally ill patients who are prone to psychological deficiencies, should again be guided by the physician into making an autonomous decision about a medical treatment. Under no circumstances is it permissible for the physician to be manipulative or coercive towards the patient. Instead, the physician has a duty to ensure that the patient's decision is rational, reflective, and autonomous.

(iii) Physicians must allow a sufficient amount of time to disclose all the relevant treatments, along with the risks and benefits involved. Disclosure of treatments is typically a time-consuming process, but the physician has a moral duty to ensure that s(he) spends as much time as is required for a patient to understand all the treatments relayed. The time required will vary from patient to patient. For some patients, the physician may need to schedule several sessions to disclose the information.

(iv) Some physicians believe they have expert knowledge that cannot be understood by the lay person. This is a faulty assumption since all technical terms have an explanation in ordinary language that can be understood to some degree by lay persons. In other words, any technical exchange can be communicated using non-technical, ordinary terminology so that it can be readily understood by the terminally ill patient. Thus, physicians should be careful and reflective about how they use language when communicating the treatments to the patient. Failure to do so may be construed as a form of manipulation since it undermines a patient's right to make a rational decision in favour or against a treatment.

(v) Personality clashes between physician and patient are not uncommon occurrences in medical situations, yet few medical professionals regard these as having a significant impact on the patient's treatment and well being. Character clashes occur when there is personal friction between physician and patient. The reasons for such a clash are usually unknown. Because of this, some physicians may feel that it is permissible to be condescending towards certain patients. This view is no doubt a backlash from the old traditional, paternalistic model of medicine in which the physician is considered as the authoritative person in the interaction. According to the paternalistic view, the physician could prescribe the treatment that s(he) believed should be administered, and the terminally ill patient should accept it. On this scheme, the terminally ill patient is treated as if s(he) is incapable of making his/her own medical decisions. However, since the early 1970's with the focus on patient autonomy, this kind of paternalistic behavior has become unacceptable. The stress on autonomy has become critical to the patient-centered approach, and the terminally ill patient's cooperation in the decision-making process with regard to a given medical treatment has become essential for an autonomous decision in favour of a medical treatment. Thus, given the current stress on partnership-based relationships between physician and patient, character clashes are not to be tolerated.

II. Shared Decision-Making

Shared decision making is the second important component for building an effective physician-patient relationship. Shared decision-making consists of: (1) acknowledging uncertainty; (2) sharing authority; (3) developing mutual trust and respect; and (4) respecting a patient's autonomy.

(1) Shared decision-making can involve the tension of uncertainty which states that physicians must not only disclose information about medical treatments, but they must also communicate any uncertainties about a medical treatment. This involves giving the terminally ill patient information about the success of a particular treatment, in addition to the possibilities that the treatment will be unsuccessful. The track record of a treatment is important for a patient to consider when making a decision in favour of or against a treatment. Terminally ill patients may choose treatments with low probabilities of success, providing they rationally decide to do so.

Physicians find it difficult to disclose uncertainties to their terminally ill patients since the medical profession is a stable science that is more or less certain to cure most illnesses, provided that they are diagnosed early. Terminally ill patients usually act on the assumption that they can completely trust medical science to cure any ailment; however, this assumption is overstated in many cases. Because of the many uncertainties that are inherent in the medical encounter, medicine should be considered to be an art that is not always free from trial and error.

(2) "Sharing authority" in decision-making does not necessarily mean that a physician and terminally ill patient must make a joint decision about a medical treatment, but instead that the patient and physician must each corroborate a decision about a medical treatment that reflects the terminally ill patient's goals, beliefs, values, and life plans. In the process of communication, the physician should guide the terminally ill patient into becoming aware of his/her deeply held beliefs, values and goals. This will ensure that the terminally ill patient will be capable of making an autonomous decision in favour of a treatment. The goal of shared decision-making is for the physician to ensure that the terminally ill patient makes an autonomous decision about a medical treatment. However, without a partnership-type relationship in which the physician and patient equally contribute to the decision-making process, an autonomous, rational, and

reflective decision about a medical treatment is difficult, if not impossible, to achieve.

Shared decision-making consists of a mutual dependency between the terminally ill patient and physician. The physician cannot disclose the information about medical alternatives without a patient's personal knowledge, and the patient cannot make a decision without an adequate disclosure of the treatments in terms that (s)he could readily understand. Thus, both the terminally ill patient and physician are considered to be an authority in different ways, in that the patient knows about his/her goals, values, beliefs, while the physician has the medical knowledge to alleviate a terminally ill patient's pain and suffering.

(3) To achieve shared decision-making, the terminally ill patient and physician must trust one other. An effective physician-patent relationship is built on trust. Due to the vulnerabilities of the medical profession and the patient's terminal illness, mutual trust is essential to fostering a relationship where the two parties can achieve open and honest communication. Mutual trust has two dimensions, one for the physician and one for the patient. The patient must trust that the physician will disclose all the information openly and honestly to ensure that (s)he can reach a rational and reflective decision in favour of a medical treatment. The physician must, in turn, trust that the patient will understand and use all the information competently and make a rational and autonomous decision in favour of a treatment.

Mutual respect between patient and physician is an essential condition for establishing an effective physician-patient relationship. Trust and respect between the terminally ill patient and physician are not easily acquired virtues. Physicians must strive to give both a diseased body and a patient's goals its proper importance and where conflicts arise, they must reconcile whether or not they will give preference to the diseased body. According to the patient-centered model, a diseased person should always take precedence over the diseased body. This presupposes that the physician must adhere to certain principles of moral behavior that respects a patient's right to self-determination.

(4) The physician must respect a terminally ill patient's autonomy by giving him/her an ample amount of time and space to make his/her own decisions about a medical treatment. Within the traditional, paternalistic model, terminally ill patients were seen as vulnerable children instead of autonomous adults. Terminal illness may weaken a patient's ability to make autonomous decisions; however, it doesn't eradicate it altogether. A patient who is chronically ill and/or in discomfort can still make autonomous decisions, although as mentioned above, the process of decision-making about a medical treatment may take considerably longer. However, the physician must not thereby conclude that the terminally ill patient is completely incapable of making an autonomous decision due to illness.

There are times that a physician may impatiently 'frame' the terminally ill patient as being incapable of autonomous decision-making, and thus proceed to either use some of the manipulative techniques discussed in this chapter, or paternalistically prescribe a treatment on behalf of the patient. Unless there is a good reason to assume that a patient really lacks a sense of self (i.e., if a patient is in a coma, unconscious, mentally challenged and so on), the physician must always assume that the patient is capable of making autonomous decisions in favour of a treatment on his/her own. Anything less, may result in erroneously undermining patient autonomy.

Conclusion

The old, traditional paternalistic model of the physician as a prescriber of medications and treatments has been dethroned. It has become a physician's implicit responsibility to ensure and assist the terminally ill patient to make autonomous, rational, reflective and well understood decisions about his/her medical treatments. This involves the practice of terminally ill patients participating in their own decision-making about medical treatments that will affect their lives, and patients must determine for themselves which medical procedures they can physically endure. On the patient-centered model, this is required in order to respect a terminally ill patient's autonomy.

Chapter 9

Advance Care Planning

The purpose of this chapter is to outline how terminally ill patients can ensure that their interests are properly represented if they become unable to do so themselves due to different levels of psychological incompetence. This chapter will address some of the moral and medical complexities that are involved in ensuring that a terminally ill patient will bring about all the advance care planning ahead of time so that his/her opinions are honoured and respected, and that abuses can be avoided. Medical professionals and relatives can sometimes bias and unfairly limit a patient's medical options. Thus, patients should enact advance care directives to protect themselves against biased judgment.

To this end, the chapter will be divided into three main parts. In Part I, I discuss two types of advance care directives that terminally ill patients enact to ensure that their autonomy will be respected. Only through advance care planning can a terminally ill patient ensure an informed consent is given for a treatment. In addition, in this chapter, I will discuss several types of advance care directives which are essential for a terminally ill patient to gain control over his/her medical treatments. In Part II, I will discuss some of the difficulties with advance directives and why the medical professionals may sometimes undervalue their authority and dishonour them. At some point, most terminally ill patients become psychologically incompetent to make important medal decisions for themselves. Part III discusses how a terminally ill patient can minimize the need for invalidating his/her advance directives. It is important that a terminally ill patient ensure that his/her advance directives are frequently revised in order for these to represent his/her current medical wishes. In this way, patient-centered care could be achieved.

I. Advance Care Directives

Advance care directives must be given top priority since a patient's self-determination is of intrinsic and instrumental value. A terminally ill patient can exercise self-determination by accepting or rejecting treatment. Thus, advance directives promote self-determination and well-being, and ensure that the terminally ill patient's interests are satisfied. Advance directives are statements that may be in written or oral form through which the terminally ill patient can control treatment decisions which arise when (s)he becomes no longer psychologically competent to do so. In order to be competent to make a medical decision, the terminally ill patient should be adequately informed and able to understand the information relevant to the treatment, and to rationally assess it in order to arrive at an autonomous choice.

Patients vary in the kind and amount of involvement they want, and perhaps need, in end-of-life decision making. Some patients prefer to enact advance directives so that their choices are respected, while others fail to do so.[1] Thus, terminally ill patients must choose the nature and extent of their involvement in end-of-life decisions. An advance directive can, therefore, take various forms, depending on the amount of detail that the patient wants to cover. In choosing the type of directives that the patient wants, (s)he is exercising self-determination in order to ensure that his/her autonomy is respected. The more detail that a terminally ill patient can provide about his/her preferences ahead of an illness, the better.

The first form of advance directive, The Values History Assessment,[2] consists of an identification of a patient's values and the articulation of advance directives based on these values. Such an assessment encourages patients to address vague issues by detailing which health care interventions should be rejected on the basis the patient's values and beliefs. The first section of the assessment encourages that the patient identify those values and beliefs which are associated with the terminal care that are most important to him/her. The goal of this overall process is to ensure that the patient becomes clear about his/her preferences, and helps physicians understand, respect, and implement the cluster of value-based decisions that were derived. The second section of the Values History Assessment begins with acute care designations: consent for or refusal of cardiopulmonary resuscitation, use of respirators, and placement of an endotracheal tube. Then, the chronic care designations follow, which include decisions for administering intravenous fluids, feeding tubes, and total parenteral nutrition for nutritional support, use of medication, and use of dialysis. Thus, the Values History Assessment gives the physician a great deal of information about the patient's beliefs, values, desires, and medical preferences.

For these reasons, the Values History Assessment should complement living wills. After the patient has signed a living will, (s)he should discuss his/her values and medical preferences with the physician, family, and relatives. First, the physician should encourage the patient to discuss his/her perspectives on the quality versus length of life. This is an important distinction that many patients resist thinking about before the onset of an illness; however, it is important for the physician to become aware of the patient's preferences. In fact, a Values History Assessment should be performed by the physician as a way of finding out more about the patient's beliefs, values, and personal and medical preferences. The Values History Assessment should also serve the purpose of making the family members aware of the patient's preferences in the event of a terminal illness. Many times, family members are unaware of the patient's specific preferences, given certain concrete medical situations, such as whether the person wants to undergo cardiopulmonary resuscitation, be placed on a ventilator, have an endoctracheal tube used or parenteral nutrition administered. By providing such information, the patient reduces familial stresses when the time comes to make such decisions.

The second form of advance directive is related to the first, except that it calls for even more detail and clarity as to the patient's preferences and aspirations, given a particular medical outcome. This statement can be beneficial for medical professionals to identify how the patient prefers to be treated, without binding that patient to the course of action, should it conflict with professional judgment. Thus, medical professionals should rely on advance directives if the course of action that a patient is proposing is contrary to what the physician perceives to be the best resolution to a patient's medical prognosis. With this form of directive, there may be instances in which the patient's autonomy will have to be overridden, if the medical situation dictates. Thus, this form of advance directive should be supplemented by other directives in order to ensure that the patient's self-determination is honoured.

The third form of advance directive consists of clear instructions refusing some or all medical procedures. If this directive is made by a competent patient, it has legal force. Some patients may leave strict instructions not to be resuscitated in certain medical situations. Other patients will leave instructions to be resuscitated, regardless of the medical situation. Still other patients will leave clear instructions not to undergo blood transfusions. Physicians have a duty to fulfill these requests since there may be legal ramifications if the physician fails to adhere to such instructions.

The fourth kind of directive is a statement that if a certain degree of irreversible deterioration occurs, no life-sustaining treatment should be administered. For instance, if a patient is in a persistent vegetative state for an extended period of time, (s)he may leave clear instructions not to be resuscitated or that (s)he should be permitted to die naturally. This directive focuses not so much on refusing a treatment as it is a request to refuse to suffer in a particular medical situation. If such a request is made by a competent patient, it has legal obligation as well. Some patients fear that they will be forced to live in a vegetative state at some point when their health deteriorates. Thus, it is essential for physicians to honor these requests.

The fifth type of directive is a written disclosure of a surrogate decision maker should the patient become unable to make a decision for him/herself. Patients must exercise caution when selecting surrogate decision makers. Many times, family members do not know a relative's best interests. In addition, abuses are possible if relatives become surrogate decision makers.[3] Thus, perhaps it would be easier for the terminally ill patient to choose a trusted friend or someone in the medical profession to represent his/her best interests when (s)he can no longer do so in a competent manner.

II. Practical Difficulties With Advance Directives

Advance directives can become invalidated by medical professionals for several reasons. First, doubts may exist about the terminally ill patient's psychological competence at the time the directives were enacted. For a directive to be valid, the patient's decision must be based on adequate information about the medical situation. The best way to achieve validity is for the patient to enact the directive at the beginning stages of a terminal illness. At that time, the patient must carefully decide how long and under which conditions (s)he is willing to endure pain and suffering. It is not necessary for the patient to enact the directive before (s)he gets ill but only before (s)he becomes incompetent. Neither is it preferable for a patient to enact the directive when the disease has progressed, since the pain and suffering may bias his/her decision. Timing is, therefore, a crucial component to enacting an effective directive.

Second, the patient must formulate the directive to cover many indeterminate ranges of medical contingencies which may be ambiguous and difficult to apply. Thus, clarity is an important prerequisite for enacting medical directives. Unless the timing is just right, there will be many ambiguities since the patient is unsure which treatments (s)he would refuse or insist upon, given his/her medical situation. It is difficult for a patient to hypothetically project how (s)he will feel about a particular situation in the future, and imagine how (s)he would want to be treated. Thus, if advance directives are enacted years before they are needed, physicians have a tendency to discredit them because they are not current portrayals of the patient's medical preferences.

Third, sometimes advance directives might relinquish self-determination, the very thing they are supposed to preserve. There are two ways that this could occur. First, when a directive is invalidated by the physician for whatever reason, a patient's self-determination is undermined. Second, when a patient enacts a directive that will not be valid, (s)he makes requests that will not represent his/her genuine needs later. Again, timing and accuracy are two essential features for enacting directives that will honour and respect a patient's autonomy when (s)he is incompetent to make his/her own medical decisions.

Fourth, competent patients are the best judges of their own character. However, serious illness can bias a patient's judgments and capacities. Thus, advance directives are time-sensitive and must be enacted neither too early nor too late. If the patient enacts the directives too early, (s)he may not be able to accurately imagine what it would be like to be in constant pain and discomfort. Thus, the directive will not fully represent his/her opinions. If the patient enacts the directives too late, the patient may not be competent to enact an effective directive. Thus, the directive may be invalidated and a surrogate may have to make decisions on behalf of the patient. It is essential that the patient choose a person that will responsibly act on his/her behalf. Otherwise, a patient's immediate family will be asked to represent his/her best interests. For this reason, physicians are skeptical about treating advance directives as genuine statements of a patient's medical preferences.

Fifth, sometimes a physician may question the authority of the advance directive. There are several reasons why advance directives do not have the same kind of authority as future contingencies. First, a patient's therapeutic options and prognosis could change between the time the directive was enacted and the time it will be implemented. A terminal disease could progress very quickly, making previous therapeutic options and treatments irrelevant. Second, the assumption that a competent patient is the best judge of his/her interests is weakened in the case of a choice about future contingencies in which the patient's overall interests could change in radical ways. The progress of a terminal illness and its effect on the patient can vary substantially over time. Again, the timing of enacting these directives is crucial to their overall validity and authority. An advance directive is not completely binding over time. Third, there are no safeguards against unreasonable choices when advance directives are enacted. Even if a choice appears unreasonable, it is not usually questioned. This makes a directive less than effective. Fourth, advance directives are often made with certain implicit assumptions in mind about the expected medical condition of the patient when a treatment option is chosen. When a patient's actual condition is substantially different, this calls into question the authority of the advance directive. It is difficult to determine how difficulties with advance directives can be avoided, or at least minimized.

III. Minimizing The Invalidation of Advance Directives

There are several ways to avoid the invalidation of directives. First, a patient should enact different kinds of directive. In this way, if one type of directive becomes invalid, the patient could rely on one of the other directives. In addition, directives should not be permanently enacted; instead, they should be revised by the patient from time to time to ensure that they accurately represent that patient's preferences. Each directive should be patient-specific and situation-specific. As a patient's medical situation changes, so will his/her preferences. Patients must ensure that their directives are accurate at all times. Each patient has a duty to enact advance directives if (s)he wants to be treated as an autonomous individual. Patients cannot expect their physicians to second-guess their preferences.

The second way to avoid invalidation is to view the directive as a work-in-progress that evolves with the patient. As a patient's medical needs change, the directives should be revised. This type of revision holds for each kind of directive. In other words, a patient could change his/her mind about his/her surrogate decision maker over time. Perhaps a patient discovered that (s)he prefers to be resuscitated in most situations, except a few. For many patients, each revised directive should bring increasing clarity. Thus, redrafts of advance directives should be encouraged by medical professionals.

Thus, when a patient's directives are periodically revised, the authority of the directive will be accurate. As a patient's therapeutic options change, (s)he must revise the directive. Also, as treatment options shift, so will the patient's overall medical goals. Perhaps prescribing more pain medication will become important to control pain for a terminally-ill patient during the last stages of his/her illness. Or, perhaps going into a hospice care facility is better than staying in a hospital or at home with an irritated spouse and relatives who feel overburdened. Such a revision of options should be written in a revised form of directive that will clearly represent a patient's interests. Such revisions will also give additional authority to the advance directive, and will ease the physician's suspicions about enacting advance directives in the first place.

Conclusion

In this chapter, I examined the importance of advance directives to ensure that a patient gives an informed consent in favour of a treatment at the end of his/her life. With advance directives, physicians will never have to second-guess their patient's preferences. Without advance directives, however, a patient's preferences will be unknown. Medical professionals should, therefore, ensure that patients do enact advance directives over the course of their lives. This is an important way for patient-centered medicine to be administered.

Chapter 10

A Humane Patient-Centered Approach to Care

The purpose of this chapter is to assess the patient-centered approach in terms of the five conditions outlined in Part II in order to achieve humane health care. As has been argued throughout the book, the patient-centered approach is especially necessary for the terminally-ill patient since many times during the last stages of a disease, such a patient is unable to mentally and/or physically make rational and effective decisions about treatment for him/herself. It is, therefore, essential that the physician ensure that the patient fulfills the five conditions of a patient-centered approach to health care. A patient has three main alternatives when (s)he becomes terminally ill. Either, the patient could choose a treatment or set of treatments which will curtail the further spread of the disease, or the patient may choose not to engage in any active treatments but to simply take pain medication until (s)he dies naturally. Lastly, the patient may choose to terminate life, if his/her medical condition becomes intolerable. Euthanasia should always be considered as a last resort. However, whichever option the terminally ill patient chooses, his/her decision must be rational, autonomous, and well thought out. If successful, the fulfillment of the five conditions of informed consent should help to ensure that a terminally ill patient makes rational decisions about end-of-life issues.

To this end, this final chapter fulfills two main purposes. First, in Part I, I will show how the patient-centered approach is necessary in administering humane health care for the terminally ill. Without personal and psychological information about the patient, the physician lacks any guidance in ensuring that a terminally ill patient gives an informed consent. A foundational component of developing a patient-centered approach is to ensure that the patient and physician feel sufficiently comfortable with each other to openly and honestly discuss the patient's medical predicament. Second, in Part II, I outline the five conditions of the patient-centered approach, the formation of an equal partnership between the patient and physician. Without the development of a partnership-type relationship, abuses can be quite prevalent among the terminally ill.

I. The Components of Humane Health Care

Humane health care for the terminally-ill involves five components. First, the physician must become increasingly sensitive to the terminally-ill patient's psychological needs and experience of illness. This is especially important since a patient has special needs that must be addressed if (s)he is to feel that his/her quality of life is not substantially reduced. Some patients may discover that they need to discuss their pain levels and fears about the future at length. Other patients have low pain thresholds, while still others will feel a lot of pain, given their unique physiological and psychological make-up. The physician must determine these pain thresholds for each patient so that (s)he can administer proper pain medication in order to keep the patient as comfortable as possible.

Secondly, the physician must become aware of some of the qualitative features that will affect the patient's life. Terminal illness usually gravely affects a patient's goals, career, and hobbies. It also can strain familial relationships and substantially restrict a patient's normal activities. It is, therefore, essential for the physician to become aware of these restrictions so that (s)he can help the patient recalibrate his/her life. Immediately after the diagnosis, the patient's family is usually too shocked to help the patient in any way that is beneficial. Thus, the physician should encourage the patient to keep doing the activities which are necessary to retain the patient's identity for as long as possible. This will also help the patient better cope with his/her terminal condition in the long-term.

Third, the physician must carefully listen to each patient's narrative of illness.[1] Every patient has a life story to which his/her illness belongs. It is part of humane health care to allow these narratives to guide medical interventions. For instance, the patient may have had a stressful life living with an abusive husband for forty years, or may have been a smoker, and overweight, all of which could have contributed to her terminal illness. It is extremely important for the physician to determine the patient's psychological and physical reasons for illness as much as possible. This will encourage the physician to determine how to best help the patient, given his/her illness.

Fourth, each patient will experience different emotions and feelings during his/her terminal illness. Some patients may become angry and depressed while others will insist on coping with the pain and hardship proactively. Some terminally-ill patients may give up on their will to live and die earlier than they should because they are afraid that their medical condition will only worsen. Thus, a physician must discuss the patient's feelings in relation to his/her terminal illness and any fears and future expectations that (s)he may have. If the physician detects that the patient is becoming depressed, (s)he should encourage the patient to speak with a counsellor. This usually encourages the patient to embrace the unknown aspects of his/her illness.

Fifth, the prognosis of every patient's illness must be assessed separately. Statistics may help the physician to achieve an overall sense of the frequency of a particular illness, given a patient's age group and life situation. However, each and every patient's life must be treated as intrinsically unique and important. A patient should never be compared to a statistic. As each patient will experience the illness differently, (s)he will endure the illness differently as well. Physicians can only roughly estimate how long a patient will live with a terminal illness. For instance, a patient's cancer may go into remission for years. Thus, it is of utmost importance that physicians treat each patient's illness as unique and somewhat unpredictable. The physician should also pay careful attention to the psychological affects of an illness since for some terminal patients, these aspects can become even more significant than the physical ones.

II. The Conditions of the Patient-Centered Approach

In this section, I will show how the five conditions of the patient-centered approach are foundational features for achieving humane health care: The five conditions are: (1) effective disclosure; (2) successful decision making; (3) effective communication; (4) developing an effective physician-patient relationship; and (5) enacting advance directives. As will be seen, there is a symmetry between the five components of humane medicine and the five conditions of the patient-centered approach. In other words, without the patient-centered approach, humane health care cannot be fully achieved.

(1) Effective disclosure and understanding between a physician-patient is essential to bring about the patient-centered approach. Ideally, a physician should openly and honestly discuss a terminally ill patient's diagnosis, prognosis, and possible treatments. Depending on the patient, the disclosure of the diagnosis, and especially the prognosis, may take two or three appointments to complete. As we saw in Chapter 4, an effective disclosure consists of several factors. The physician must foster an understanding of the patient's medical predicament by trying to ascertain, along with the patient, how the illness will psychologically and physically affect the patient's overall life. A physician can achieve this by becoming sensitive to the patient's needs and experience of illness.

(2) Since the terminally ill patient is initially shocked after a negative diagnosis, (s)he may not be able to make a rational, reflective decision which avoids erroneous cognitive biases. Thus, the physician must encourage the patient to make a rational and informed decision in favour of a treatment. The

physician must view the terminally ill patient as a unique person, with special needs and vulnerabilities. The patient, on the other hand, must regard the physician as an individual who can guide him/her to make an informed consent, if necessary, by ensuring that (s)he makes a decision in favour of or against a treatment that coheres with his/her long-term goals and values. If the decision is out of character, the physician should guide the terminally ill patient by reminding him/her of his/her long-term goals and values. Without shared decision-making, a terminally ill patient may make an irrational decision in favour of or against a treatment.

(3) A physician must effectively communicate the diagnosis, prognosis, and treatment options to the patient. Within the patient-centered approach, this is achieved by focusing on the patient's narrative of illness. In other words, after the diagnosis, prognosis, and treatment options are disclosed, the physician must carefully listen to the terminally ill patient. A patient's life is usually disrupted and (s)he is confused because of the illness. Nothing seems to be the way it used to be. The terminally ill patient may feel increasingly weak and in constant pain. Further, the treatments may not initially be helping but merely causing a lot of negative side effects.Thus, a terminally ill patient's experience of illness must be taken into consideration in order to treat him/her in a humane manner.

In addition, the treatments must be disclosed clearly so that they are properly understood by the patient. When a terminally ill patient is in shock, (s)he will not be able to make a rational decision in favour or against a medical treatment since (s)he will feel hopeless and might bias the decision to be made. Some patients may need to spend a substantial amount of time with their physicians discussing their fears. Once the initial shock has subsided, the patient will be enacted to make a rational decision about a medical treatment. During this time, the physician should become aware of the terminally ill patient's overall feelings towards his/her diagnosis and prognosis.

Without a complete open and honest disclosure of the diagnosis, prognosis, and treatments, the terminally ill patient cannot give an informed consent for or against a treatment. The physician must also disclose all the risks that are involved for a particular treatment. If the physician does not know if a particular treatment will be beneficial for the terminally ill patient, (s)he should disclose such uncertainties to the patient. Further, the physician should also disclose the success rates of certain procedures based on past records. This may encourage a terminally ill patient to feel more hopeful and confident about the treatment.

The traditional paradigm of medicine views the patient's illness as a diseased body that could be cured by relying on various kinds of treatment and/or surgery. For the physician, a disease state is an entity that can be separated from the patient experiencing the illness. According to the patient-centered approach, the illness is part of his/her body and substantially affects the patient's quality of life since it adversely affects his/her sense of personhood. The difference between the physician's narrative of illness as a disease and the patient's as a lived experience highlights the reason why the patient and physician often discover how difficult it is to effectively communicate with one another. The five conditions of the patient-centered approach advocated throughout the book propose ways to break the barriers to effective communication.

In order to help the patient cope with the disruption of a terminal illness, the physician must shift focus from the diseased state of a patient's body to the lived experience of the illness. This shift in focus requires a phenomenological analysis of the illness. When a physician interprets a terminal-illness as a diseased state, s(he) objectifies the patient and in the process separates him/her from his/her body and self. However, the patient's body and self are intrinsic aspects of the terminal illness, and a physician cannot effectively prescribe treatments without treating both the patient's body and the mind. This presupposes that the physician must pay particular attention to the psychological and physical disturbances that the patient is experiencing as a result of his/her terminal illness. In other words, it is essential that the physician shift his/her focus from the objective features of disease to the subjective, personal features of the terminal illness during the clinical encounter. Physicians must, therefore, spend a considerable amount of time during the clinical encounter discussing the impact that a particular terminal illness will have on a patient's quality of life. Many times the physician will have to reassure the patient by encouraging him/her to endure and persevere during the illness, and by helping him/her gain the strength to resume his/her normal daily activities and long and short-term projects. Thus, the physician may have to heal the patient both psychologically and physically since terminal illness manifests itself both ways.[2]

In addition, the subjective meaning can most accurately be known by the terminally ill patient experiencing it. This does not mean that the terminally ill patient cannot express the pain s(he) is experiencing in a way that can be understood by the physician. A patient understands what an illness means, when s(he) determines how important it is in his/her personal life. This sense of meaning presupposes a unique kind of particularity. For instance, when a terminally ill patient experiences severe pain for the first time, the patient's narrative will be subjective in that s(he) will report on the particular effects that the pain has had on his/her body, mind, and long and short-term goals. The terminally ill patient may say, "I couldn't participate in a walkaton for MS this year"; or "I haven't exercised for six months"; or "I haven't been able to go to work for the last few weeks". These narrative reports highlight the subjective effects of the terminal illness on the patient's life. This sense of the subjective is essential for the physician in achieving an effective diagnosis and treatment for illness.

This shift in perspective from objective to subjective must be extended into the clinical encounter between a physician-patient in order for the physician and patient to communicate effectively. According to the patient-centered approach, the physician must listen carefully to the patient's verbal reports and avowals of illness so that s(he) can determine the patient's fears and anxieties about the illness, and how his/her life will be disrupted. On the basis of such information, the physician can then proceed to use proper diagnostic procedures to suggest treatments. A diagnosis is most often achieved through laboratory tests (such as blood tests, x-rays, urine samples), stethoscope, EEG's and so on, all of which are objective measures that diagnose the patient's illness. In this way, the physician can both heal and cure the patient.

It is important to note that the clinical narrative is distinct from the patient's medical history which consists of the patient's state of health over his/her whole life. A patient's medical history consists of facts about symptoms, disease etiology, and potential for treatment. The clinical narrative, on the other hand, provides insights about how an illness affects the narrative of the patient which is the patient's story of illness. The clinical narrative may be less precise than the patient's perspective; however, it is especially relevant to the medical diagnosis and treatment of a terminal illness. The physician must, therefore, spend a significant amount of time after the diagnosis examining the clinical narrative and the medical history of the terminally ill patient.

According to the patient-centered approach, a clinical narrative has both psychological and physical features. Both features are communicated through the terminally ill patient. Patients are not merely objective observers reporting on their illness; they can also tell the physician the personal symptoms of their illness, and the impact it has on their lives. Thus, by attending to the experiential aspects of terminal illness, the physician can effectively understand how the patient is experiencing his/her illness. The clinical narrative discloses what it is like for a particular patient to be suffering from a particular terminal illness. The clinical narrative is, therefore, beneficial for the physician in understanding the patient's suffering. This process will also ensure that the physician will empathize with the patient and determine what it is like for a patient to be suffering from a particular illness, given his/her narrative history. Through empathy, the physician can prescribe treatments that will be most beneficial to the patient's terminal illness and his/her unique experience of the illness. This is an essential aspect of humane medicine.

(4) One method of developing an effective physician-patient relationship is by fostering shared understanding, which is based on a reciprocal understanding between patient and physician. Ordinary understanding substantially differs from reciprocal understanding since the former consists of the physician merely communicating the facts of the available treatments to the patient whereas the latter takes the patient's personal needs and values into consideration. According to the patient-centered approach, it is insufficient for the physician to communicate the facts of the treatments without personalizing them to the

patient's needs, values, goals, and long and short-term beliefs. The personal features of the treatments must be determined through shared understanding.

Without shared understanding and mutual trust and respect, an open, honest physician-patient relationship cannot be developed. Because of the inherent vulnerabilities of the terminally ill patient, the physician must understand and empathize with the terminally ill patient's predicament for humane medicine to be achieved. This recognition should facilitate the physician's understanding and hopefully lead to reciprocal understanding. The physician must, therefore, always facilitate an open, honest dialogue through which a patient's fears are openly discussed and uncertainties of treatment and prognosis communicated.

(5) Shared understanding is especially important for advance care planning. In many cases, the physician should encourage the terminally ill patient to enact advance directives, ideally before (s)he is incapacitated by the terminal illness. It is advised that a terminally ill patient not merely determine who will exercise his/her power of attorney but enact a living will and advance directives, laying out his/her medical orders should (s)he be unable to make medical decisions in the future. The directives should include whether the patient wants to be kept alive, regardless of his/her psychological prognosis or not resuscitated in certain clearly defined circumstances.

Thus, within the patient-centered approach, the terminally ill patient and physician must form an equal partnership. The physician cannot determine the terminally ill patient's beliefs, values, and goals on his/her own without consulting the patient. The terminally ill patient, on the other hand, needs the physician to provide the medical knowledge that is necessary to help the patient cope with the illness. The physician should also ensure that the terminally ill patient gives an informed consent for a procedure, if (s)he is aware of the patient's beliefs, values, and long and short-term goals. Further, the longer a terminally ill patient endures pain and discomfort, the more vulnerable will (s)he feel. The physician will need to both psychologically and physically support the terminally ill patient.

In addition, medical professionals and relatives can sometimes bias and unfairly limit a terminally ill patient's options. Thus, patients should enact advance care directives to protect themselves against biased judgment and to uphold a patient-centered approach to medicine. For this reason, advance care directives must be given top priority since a patient's self-determination is of intrinsic value. A terminally ill patient can exercise self-determination by accepting or rejecting treatment now and in the future. Thus, advance directives promote self-determination and well-being, and ensure that the terminally ill patient's interests are satisfied. Humane medicine is achieved by ensuring that a patient's future wishes are upheld.

Conclusion

The importance of the five conditions which define the patient-centered approach to medicine for the terminally ill cannot be overestimated. Without these conditions, the patient usually cannot decide on the treatments which are best for him/her. Usually, the terminally ill patient is at the mercy of relatives or health professionals who know very little about the patient. Many times, a terminally ill patient's life is ended against his/her will. One way that the physician could ensure that a terminally ill patient gives an informed consent is by adhering to the five components of humane medicine and the five conditions outlined in Part II of the book.

Notes

Chapter 1

1. See Kenneth A. Richman's Ethics and the Metaphysics of Medicine: Reflections on Health and Beneficence. (Cambridge, Massachussetts: The MIT Press, 2004), p. 162-163.
2. See Francis W. Peabody. The Care of the Patient. (Cambridge, Massachusetts: Harvard University Press, 1927).
3. I say 'ideally' because there are situations in which the physician only meets the patient at the onset of a terminal illness. However, in such situations, I believe that there is still ample time to get to know the patient.

Chapter 2

1. See Ezekiel J. Emanuel and Linda L. Emanuel's "Four Models of the Physician Patient Relationship", in *The Journal of the American Medical Association,* 267(16), (1992), 2221-2226.
2. See "Four Models of the Physician-Patient Relationship".
3. See Richard M. Frankel, Timothy E. Quill, Susan H. McDaniel's, *The Biopsychosocial Approach: Past, Present, Future.* New York: The University of Rochester Press, 2003.
4. See "Four Models of the Physician-Patient Relationship".
5. See Earl. E. Shelp's, *The Clinical Encounter: The Moral Fabric of the Patient-Physician Relationship.* Dordrecht: D. Reidel Publishing Company, 1983.
6. 'Benevolent Paternalism' is characterized by Emanuel, Emanuel as 'Paternalism' in "Four Models of the Physician-Patient Relationship", p. 2221.

7. The Customer-salesperson model is characterized by Emanuel, Emanuel as "The Informative Model", in "Four Models of the Physician-Patient Relationship", p. 2221.
8. The "Contractual Model" is outlined in *The Biopsychosocial Approach: Past, Present, Future,* p. 44.
9. The Partnership Model is characterized by Emanuel and Emanuel as the 'Interpretive Model' in "Four Models of the Physician-Patient Relationship", p. 2221-2222.
10. See Earl. E. Shelp's, *The Clinical Encounter: The Moral Fabric of the Patient-Physician Relationship,* Chapter 4.

Chapter 3

1. I realize that it is not the norm for physicians to short-shrift a patient's aspirations in this way. However, the point I am making is that a terminally ill patient should be encouraged to do whatever (s)he aspires to if that is possible before (s)he becomes terminally ill.
2. This is especially the case for patients who become terminally ill in their middle years.

Chapter 4

1. Balint, M., Hunt, I., Joyce, D., Marinker, M., and Woodcock, J. *Treatment or Diagnosis: a Study of Repeat Prescriptions in General Practice,* (Philadelphia: J.B. Lippincott, 1970).
2. See Wright, H.I. and MacAdam, D.B. *Clinical Thinking and Practice: Diagnosis and Decision in Patient Care.* (Edinburgh, Scotland: Churchill Livingstone, 1979).
3. In this paper, I will argue in favour of the patient-centered approach since I believe that the four conditions essentially rely on the patient-centered approach in order to bring about humane health care for the terminally-ill patient.
4. See Moira Stewart, Judith Belle Brown, Wayne Weston, Ian R. McWhinney, Carol L. McWilliam, and Thomas R. Freeman's *Patient-Centered Medicine: Transforming the Clinical Method,* (London: Sage Publications, 1995), p. 27ff.
5. See Stewart's et al's *Patient-Centered Medicine,* p. 28.
6. Ibid., p. 1.
7. See K. Toombs, *The Meaning of Illness: A Phenomenological Account of the Different Perspectives of Physician and Patient.* (Norwell, M.A.: Kluwer Publishing, 1992).
8. See Arthur Frank's *At the Will of the Body: Reflection on Illness,* (Boston: Houghton Miffin, 1991), p. 48.

9. Lowenstein, Jerome. The Midnight Meal and Other Essays about Doctors, Patients, and Medicine. (Ann Arbor: The University of Michigan Press, 2005), p. 122.
10. Lowenstein, p. 106.
11. Lowenstein, p. 107.
12. Lowenstein, p. 68ff.

Chapter 5

1. I will delve into these concepts more specifically later.
2. Honesty is objective because it can be measured and little is left to individual choice. The honesty of a physician's diagnosis could be determined by other individuals. If a physician discloses all aspects of the diagnosis (even the uncertainties), (s)he is providing an honest diagnosis. If a physician only discloses the test results that (s)he believes that the patient will want to hear, the physician is dishonest with his/her disclosure and disrespects the patient. In addition, dishonesty does not contribute to effective communication. To communicate with a patient effectively, the physician must respect the patient's autonomy. Lastly, if a physician fails to disclose any aspect of the diagnosis, (s)he is dishonest. This is unacceptable under any circumstances, especially in the situation of a terminal illness since each patient has a right to know whether or not (s)he has a terminal disease as soon as it is detected. The physician has no choice but to disclose the diagnosis, regardless of what (s)he thinks about how the patient will handle the diagnosis.
3. See Irene Switankowsky's A New Paradigm For Informed Consent (Lanham, Maryland: University Press of America, 1997), Chapter 4, p. 59.
4. It should be noted that these three conditions do not exhaust all the conditions which are necessary for a terminally ill patient to understand all the medical alternatives disclosed to him/her.
5. I realize that not all families are in this predicament. Some families communicate honestly with one another. However, upon examining the literature, it is safe to say that this is the exception rather than the rule.

Chapter 6

1. Individuals who are incapable of engaging in a sufficient degree of reflection required for rational decisions will be excluded from this study. On the autonomy-enhancing model, the rationality that an informed consent demands as a necessary condition is beyond such individuals' emotional and intellectual capability. In short, patients who do not have a coherent picture of the self will find it very difficult to make autonomous, rational and informed decisions. It is not the responsibility of physicians to guide such patients into forming a

coherent set of beliefs and values. This is definitely beyond the physician's call of duty and perhaps even beyond the call of a psychologist.

2.   It may be useful to note that there are merely four systems of belief (although there may be a few others) outlined in Figure 5.1, and many network beliefs (again, only a few of which are outlined). There is also an overlap of the network beliefs. In figure 5.1 and 5.2, 'duty bound', 'honesty', and 'reflectiveness' appears in the 'religious' and 'moral' system beliefs. This is typically the way an individual's system beliefs overlap. My intention here is to give the reader a general idea as to how we could determine our belief systems and their networks. Hopefully, this will facilitate understanding of this somewhat vague section of the chapter. Some of the epistemological jargon used here originates from Keith Lehrer's *Theory of Knowledge*, although I depart from his account by excluding some of the theoretical aspects of his epistemological theory for ease of understanding by the lay person who is untouched by epistemology and/or philosophy. Lehrer distinguishes between systems and ultra systems. I merely refer to belief-systems and networks of belief.

3. The number of treatments derived is unimportant. It must only be a manageable number so that the patient does not reach cognitive-information overload.

4.   Kahneman and Tversky wrote several articles on 'biases' and 'heuristics'. Some of the more relevant ones for my purposes are: (1) Kahneman, Daniel, & Tversky, Amos. "Choices, Frames and Values". *American Psychologist*, 1984, Volume 39(4), 341-350. (2) Kahneman, Daniel & Tversky, Amos. "Judgment Under Uncertainty: Heuristics and Biases". *Science*, (1974) 125, 1124-1131. (3) Tversky, A., and Kahneman, D. "The Framing of Decisions and the Psychology of Choice". *Science*, 211, 453-458.

Chapter 7

1. Honesty in medical contexts is an important problem. The following articles are only a sample of the debate currently in progress:

    Jackson, Jennifer. "Telling The Truth". *Journal of Medical Ethics*, 17 (1991), 5-9.

    Minogue, Brendan, P., & Taraszewski. "The Whole Truth and Nothing But The Truth?" *Hastings Center Report*, (October-November, 1988), 34-36.

2. Michael Lockwood. *Moral Dilemmas in Modern Medicine*, chapter on "The Truth" by Roger Higgs, p. 187-202.

3. Lockwood, p. 190.

4. Sometimes deception is characterized in terms of lying. However, I argue that the two terms have distinct meanings because even though the terms aim at a similar result (being dishonest to a patient), their intention has different degrees

and intensities. Lying is a much more direct form of dishonesty than deception which may be considered indirect. Furthermore, deception is often considered justified by some physicians in some circumstances.

5. In this section, I will first focus on the physician's responsibility to keep information confidential because it is my contention that there is a greater tendency for the physician to disclose confidential information to other third parties than for the patient to do so. Thus, the discussion will seem unequally balanced.

6. The only condition under which physicians could disclose information about the patient to the nursing staff or any other medical practitioners is if such individuals are directly responsible for the medical treatment of the patient. Even in those cases, the patient should be explicitly aware to whom the information is disclosed. However, no information about the patient should be disclosed to any other individuals without the patient's express permission.

Chapter 8

1. Psychological competency in this case means intelligence and emotional perspicuity.

2. For further discussion on the tension of authority see Steven Katz's *The Silent World of Doctor and Patient*.

Chapter 9

1. See Fiona Randall's and R.S. Downie's *Palliative Care Ethics: A Companion for All Specialties* (Oxford: Oxford University Press, 2002), pg. 191ff.

2. For a copy of a Value History Assessment, see David J. Doukas and Laurence B. McCullough's "The Values History: The Evaluation of the Patient's Values and Advance Directives", *The Journal of Family Practice*, (1991), Vol. 32(2), 151-153.

3. See Dan W. Brock's "Good Decision-Making for Incompetent Patients," in *The Hastings Center Report, Special Supplement*, November-December, 1994, S8-S11.

Chapter 10

1. The patient may have had to work hard all his/her life. Or, the patient may have had to endure physical and/or psychological stress during his/her thirty-year marriage. Or, the patient may have been a smoker and didn't exercise most of his/her life. All of these narratives will help the physician treat the patient's illness uniquely in accordance to his/her personal needs.

2. The subjective components involve understanding the personal meaning an illness has for the patient. Discussions about subjective medical information in the literature tend to collapse the distinction between the subjectivity of the patient and the subjectivity of the physician. In the following, I will only be concerned with patient subjectivity in the clinical encounter. There are at least two possible meanings of 'subjective' in this context. First, 'subjective' may mean a perception of a state of affairs that is relative to the particular terminally ill patient. This makes his/her avowals idiosyncratic and inexpressible to their parties without careful attention. This meaning of 'subjective' will not concern me as I believe that the physician can adequately understand the terminally ill patient's avowals since they share a common language. The second meaning of 'subjective' involves the inner states or bodily sensations of a patient. These avowals consist of qualitative reports of bodily sensations such as nausea, pain, aches, and so on. These symptomatic reports comprise the clinical narrative of the patient.

Bibliography

Abu-Saad, Huda.*Evidence-Based Palliative Care: Across the Life Span.* Oxford: Blackwell Sciences Ltd., 2001.

Aring, Charles, D. "Sympathy and Empathy". *The Journal of the American Medical Association.* Volume 167(4), 1958, 448-452.

Baird, Robert, M., Rosenbaum, Stuart E. *Caring for the Dying: Critical Issues at the Edge of Life.* Amherst, New York: Prometheus Books, 2000.

Barnard, David, Towers, Anna, Boston, Patricia, Lambrinidou, Yanna.*Crossing Over: Narratives of Palliative Care.* Oxford: Oxford University Press, 2000.

Beauchamp, T., & Childress, J. *Principles of Biomedical Ethics.* New York: Oxford University Press, 1979.

Bertakis, Klea, D., Roter, Debra, Putnam, Samuel, M. "The Relationship of Physician Medical Interview Style to Patient Satisfaction". *The Journal of Family Practice,* 32(2), (1991), 175-181.

Brock, Dan. W. "Good Decisionmaking for Incompetent Patients". *Special Supplement: Hastings Center Report.* November-December, (1994), S8-S10.

Brown, Betz, Jonathan, Boles, Myde, Mullooly, John, P., Levinson, Wendy. "Effect of Clinician Communication Skills Training on Patient Satisfaction". *Annals of Internal Medicine,* 131(11), (1999), 822-829.

Buller, Mary Klein, Buller, David, B. "Physicians' Communication Style and Patient Satisfaction." *Journal of Health and Behavior.* Volume 28, (1987), 375-388.

Glumgart, Hermann, L. "Caring For the Patient". *The New England Journal of Medicine.* Volume 270(9), (1964), 444-456.

Brody, Howard. *Stories of Sickness.* New Haven and London: Yale University Press, 1987.

Brody, Howard. *The Healer's Power.* New Haven and London: Yale University Press, 1992.

Brody, H. "Transparency: Informed Consent in Primary Care".*Hastings Centre Report.* Volume 19, (1989), 5-9.

Bennett, Henry, L. "Trees and Heads: The Objective and the Subjective in Painful Procedures". *The Journal of Clinical Ethics,* 5(3), (1994), 149-151.

Buchanan, Allen, B. *Deciding for Others: The Ethics of Surrogate Decision Making.* New York: Cambridge University Press, 1992.

Buehler, David, A. "Informed Consent - Wishful Thinking?"*Journal of Medical and Human Bioethics.* Volume 4, (1982), 43-57.

Cassell, Eric, J. *The Healer's Art: A New Approach to the Doctor-Patient Relationship.* Philadelphia and New York: J.B. Lippincott Company, 1998.

Cassell, Eric, J. "The Function of Medicine". *Hastings Center Report,* (1977), 16-19.

Coleman, Lester, L. "The Patient-Physician Relationship", in *Physician'sWorld,* 1974.

Danis, Marion. "Following Advance Directives". *Special Supplement: Hastings Center Report.* November-December, (1994), S21-S23.

Ditto, Peter, H., Coppola, Kristen, M., Houts, Renate, M. "Advance Directives as Acts of Communication. *Archives of Internal Medicine,* 161, (2001), 421-430.

Doukas, David, J., McCullough, Laurence, B. "The Evaluation of the Patient's Values and Advance Directives". *The Journal of Family Practice,* Vol. 32(2) (1991), 145-154.

Dresser, Rebecca. "Advance Directives: Implications for Policy". *Special Supplement: Hastings Center Report.* November-December, (1994), S2-S5.

Dworkin, Gerald, Frey, R.G., Bok, Sissela. *Euthanasia and Physician- Assisted Suicide: For and Against.* Cambridge: Cambridge University Press, 1998.

Elias, Sherman, & Annas, George, J. "The Whole Truth and Nothing But the Truth?" *Hastings Centre Report,* Volume 18, (1988), 35-36.

Emanuel, Ezekiel, J. & Emanuel, Linda, L. "The Medical Directive."*Journal of The American Medical Association.* Volume 261(22), (1989), 3288-3293.

Emanuel, Ezekiel, J. & Emanuel, Linda, L. "Four Models of the Physician-Patient Relationship". *Journal of American Medical Association,* 267(16), (1992), 2221-2226.

Emanuel, Ezekiel, J. & Emanuel, Linda, L. "Decisions at the End of Life: Guided by Communities of Patients". *Hastings Center Report,* September-October, (1993), 6-14

Emanuel, Linda. "What Makes a Directive Valid?" *Special Supplement: Hastings Center Report.* November-December, (1994), S27-S28.

Faden, Ruth, R., & Beauchamp, Tom L. *A History and Theory of Informed Consent.* New York: Oxford University Press, 1986.

Forrow, Lachlan. "The Green Eggs and Ham Phenomena". *Special Supplement: Hastings Center Report.* November to December, (1994), S29-S32.

Fromer, Margot, Joan. *Ethical Issues in Health Care.* St.Louis:Mosby, 1981.

Hackler, Chris, Moseley, Ray, Vawter, Dorothy, E. *Advance Directives in Medicine.* New York: Praeger Publishers, 1989.

Hall, Judith, A., Dornan, Michael, C. "What Patients Like About their Medical Care and How Often They Are Asked: A Meta-Analysis of the Satisfaction Literature". *Social Science and Medicine,* 27(9), (1988), 935-939.

Hendin, Herbert. "Selling Death and Dignity". *Hastings Center Report,* May-June, (1995), 6-12.

Heinz, Donald. *The Last Passage: Recovering a Death of Our Own.* Oxford: Oxford University Press, 1999.

High, Dallas, M. "Families' Roles in Advance Directives". *Special Supplement: Hastings Center Report.* November-December, (1994), S16-S18.

Jackson, Jennifer. "Telling The Truth". *Journal of Medical Ethics,* 17 (1991), 5-9.

Kahneman, Daniel, & Tversky, Amos. "Choices, Frames and Values". *American Psychologist,* (1984), Volume 39(4), 341-350.

Kantor, Jay, E. *Medical Ethics for Physicians-in-Training.* New York: Plenum Medical Book Company, 1989.

Katz, Jay. *The Silent World of Doctor and Patient.* New York: Free Press, 1984.

Kleespies, Phillip, M. *Life and Death Decisions: Psychological and Ethical Considerations in End-of-Life Care.* Washington, D.C.: American Psychological Association, 2004.

Kohut, Nitsa, Sam, Mehran, O'Rourke, Keith, MacFadden, Douglas, K., Salit, Irving, Singer, Peter, A. "Stability of Treatment Preferences: Although Most Preferences do not Change, Most People Change Some of Their Preferences". *Journal of Clinical Ethics.* Volume 8(2), (1997), 124-135.

Lee, Melinda, A., Smith, David, M., Fenn, Darien, S., Ganzini, Linda. "Do Patients' Treatment Decisions Match Advance Statements of Their Preferences? *Journal of Clinical Ethics.* Volume 9(3), (1998), 258-262.

Lewis, Rees, J. "Patient Views on Quality Care in General Practice: Literature Review". *Social Science and Medicine,* 39(5), (1994), 655-670.

Like, Robert, Zyzanski, Stephen. "Patient Satisfaction with the Clinical Encounter: Social Psychological Determinants". *Social Science and Medicine,* 24(4), (1987), 351-357.

Lindemann, Nelson, Hilde, Lindemann Nelson James. "Preferences and Other Moral Sources". *Special Supplement: Hastings Center Report.* November-December, (1994), S19-S20.

Lowenstein, Jerome. *The Midnight Meal and Other Essays about Doctors, Patients, and Medicine.* Ann Arbor: The University of Michigan Press, 2005.

McCullough, Laurence, & Christianson, Charles. "Ethical Dimensions of Diagnosis". *Metamedicine*, (1981), Vol. 2, 129-141.

Miles, Steven, H. "Physician-Assisted Suicide and the Profession's Gyrocompass". *Hastings Center Report*. May-June, (1995), 17-19.

Minogue, Brendan, P., & Taraszewski. "The Whole Truth and Nothing But The Truth?" *Hastings Center Report*, October-November, (1988), 34-36.

Morreim, Haavi. "Three Concepts of Patient Competence". *Theoretical Medicine*, 4 (1983), 231-252.

Niemira, Denise. "Life on the Slippery Slope: A Bedside View of Treating Incompetent Elderly Patients". *Hastings Center Report,* May-June, (1993), 14-17.

Novack, Dennis, H., Detering, Barbara, J., Arnold, Robert, Forrow, Lachlan, Landinsky, Morissa, & Pezullo, John, C. "Physicians' Attitudes Toward Using Deception to Resolve Difficult Ethical Problems". *Journal of American Medical Association*, 261(20), (1989), 2980-2985.

Paasche-Orlow, Michael, Roter, Debra. "The Communication Patterns of Internal Medicine and Family Practice Physicians". *The Journal of theAmerican Board of Family Practice,* 16, (2003), 485-493.

Payne, Sheila, Ellis-Hill, Caroline. *Chronic and Terminal Illness: New Perspectives on Caring and Careers.* Oxford: Oxford University Press, 2001.

Pearlman, Allan, Robert. "Are We Asking the Right Questions". *Special Supplement: Hastings Center Report.* November-December, (1994), S24-S27.

Ptacek, J.T., Eberhardt, Tara, L. "Breaking Bad News: A Review of the Literature". *The Journal of the American Medical Association,* 276(6), (1996), 496-502.

Quill, Timothy, E.*Caring for Patients At the End-of- Life: Facing an Uncertain Future together.* Oxford: Oxford University Press, 2001.

Randall, Fiona, Downie, R.S. *Palliative Care Ethics: A Companion For All Specialties.* Oxford: Oxford University Press, 1999.

Resnik, David, B., Rehm, Marsha, Minard, Raymond, B. "The Undertreatment of Pain: Scientific, Clinical, Cultural, and Philosophical Factors". *Medicine, Health care and Philosophy,* 4, (2001), 277-288.

Robertson, John. A. "Second Thoughts on Living Wills". *Hastings Center Report,* November-December, (1991), 6-9.

Robbins, Dennis, A. *Ethical Dimensions of Clinical Medicine.* Springfield: Thomas, 1981.

Rosenberg, James, E., & Toweres, Bernard. "The Practice of Empathy as a Prerequisite for Informed Consent". *Theoretical Medicine, 7* (1986), 181-194.

Sachs, Greg, A. "Increasing the Prevalence of Advance Care Planning: *Special Supplement: Hastings Center Report.* November-December, (1994), S13-S15.

Scofield, Giles, R. "Is Consent Useful When Resuscitation Isn't"? *Hastings Center Report,* November-December, (1991), 28-36.

Shelp, Earl. E. *The Clinical Encounter: The Moral Fabric of the Patient-Physician Relationship.* Dordrecht: D. Reidel Publishing Company, 1983.

Smith, David, H. *Respect and Care in Medical Ethics.* Lanham: University Press of America, 1985.

Spiro, Howard M., Curnen Mccrea, Mary G. *Empathy and the Practice of Medicine: Beyond Pills and Scapel.* New Haven: Yale University Press, 1993.

Stewart, Moira. "What is a Successful Doctor-Patient Interview? A Study of Interactions and Outcomes?" *Social Science and Medicine,* 19(2), (1984), 167-175.

Stewart, Moira, Brown, Judith Belle, Weston, Wayne, E., McWhinney, Ian R., McWilliam Carol, L., Freeman, Thomas, R. *Patient-Centered Medicine: Transforming The Clinical Method.* London: Sage Publications, 1995.

Suchman, Anthony, L., Markakis, Kathryn, Beckman, Howard, B., Frankel, Richard. A Model of Empathic Communication in the Medical Interview. *Journal of the American Medical Association.* Vol. 277(8), (1997), 678-682.

Sugarman, Jeremy. "Recognizing Good Decisionmaking for Incapacitated Patients". *Special Supplement: Hastings Center Report.* November-December, (1994), S11-S13.

Ten Have, Henk, AMJ, Welie, Jos, V.M. "Euthanasia: Normal Medical Practice? *Hastings Center Report.* 1992, 34-38.

Teno, Joan, M., Lindemann, Nelson, Hilde, Lynn Joanne. "AdvanceCare Planning: Priorities for Ethical and Empirical Research". *Special Supplement: Hastings Center Report.* November-December, 1994, S32-S36.

Thom, David, H., Campbell, Bruce. "Patient-Physician Trust: An Exploratory Study". *The Journal of Family Practice,* 44(2), (1997), 169-176.

Tversky, Amos. "Elimination by Aspects". *Psychological Review.* Volume 79(4), (1972), 281-299.

Tversky, Amos, & Kahneman, Daniel. "The Framing of Decisions and the Psychology of Choice". *Science,* Volume 211, (1981), 453-458.

Tversky, Amos, & Kahneman, Daniel. "Judgment Under Uncertainty". *Science,* Volume 85, (1974), 1124-1131.

Veatch, Robert, M. "Abandoning Informed Consent". *Hastings Center Report,* March-April, (1995), 5-12.

Veatch, Robert, M. *A Theory of Medical Ethics.* New York: Basic Books, Inc., 1981.

Veatch, Robert, M. "Why Get Consent?" *Hospital Physician*. Volume 11, (1975), 30-31.

Wear, Stephen. *Informed Consent: Patient Autonomy and Clinician Beneficence Within Health Care.* Washington, D.C.: Georgetown University Press, 1998.

Welie, Jos, V.M., Welie, Sander, P.K. "Patient decision Making Competence: Outlines of a Conceptual Analysis". *Medicine, Health Care and Philosophy,* 4, (2001), 127-138.

Welie, Sander, P.K. "Criteria For Patient Decision Making (In)Competence: A Review of and Commentary on Some Empirical Approaches". *Medicine, Health Care and Philosophy,* 4, (2001), 139-151.

Wetle, Terrie. "Individual Preferences and Advance Directives". *Special Supplement: Hastings Center Report.* November-December, (1994), S5-S7.

Wright, Richard, A. *Human Values in Health Care: The Practice of Ethics.* New York: McGraw Hill, 1988.